A JOURNEY TO PEACE
THROUGH YOGA

Published by Brolga Publishing Pty Ltd
PO Box 12544 A'Beckett St Melbourne Australia 8006
ABN 46 063 962 443
email: sales@brolgapublishing.com.au
web: www.brolgapublishing.com.au

National Library of Australia Cataloguing-in-Publication entry:

    Dickinson, Lynnette.
    A journey to peace through yoga / Lynnette Dickinson.
    9781921596797 (pbk.)
    Dickinson, Lynnette.
    Yoga—Therapeutic use.
    Meditation—Therapeutic use.
    Multiple sclerosis—Australia—Patients—Biography.
    Multiple sclerosis—Australia—Patients—Attitudes.
    362.1968340092

Printed in Indonesia
Cover design by David Khan
Typesetting by Takiri Nia

A JOURNEY TO PEACE THROUGH YOGA

Lynnette Dickinson

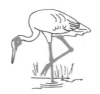

Dedicated to

Gabriel, Grace and Nicola
Who have given me a reason to go on when I didn't think
I could and taught me how to love.

With thanks to

My teachers and their teachers,
through the lineage of Dru
The classes of CNO7 & DM08
All of the carers and health professionals who
have given me such care
My family
And Matthew, who told me I could.

FOREWORD

From wheelchair to walking in under a year? Even as a seasoned observer of yoga's tremendous health benefits, I wouldn't have thought it likely that someone could use yoga to make such a dramatic change in their health in such a short time.

However, that is just one of the achievements Lynnette Dickinson describes in this outstanding book. And remarkably, Lynnette leaves a clear trail others can use to replicate her achievement. Her story will make you laugh, it will make you cry, but most importantly, Lynnette's chronicle of her challenges, her triumphs, and the methods that she used make it possible for others to benefit so much by following her example.

Most readers will be familiar with Marianne Williamson's famous statement quoted in Nelson Mandela's inauguration address that 'it is our light, not our darkness, that is our deepest fear.'

Lynnette has confronted this fear, accepted it, and then gone on to overcome it with truly lightning speed.

When I first sat with Lynnette for an in-depth conversation she was bound in a wheelchair by the debilitating effects of MS. She clearly managed heroically, every day, to give magnificently to her family, her friends, and her students. Yet as our conversation unfolded I began to suspect that she was also bound by a mental-emotional state of denying that giving to herself.

All my experience led me to be confident that yoga could help her make a difference. I've seen victims of war use yoga techniques to heal emotional traumas in conflict zones in Africa and Europe. Most yoga techniques can be done by any person, of any physical ability, from any culture, and I knew we would be able to adapt Lynnette's yoga to a wheelchair environment.

But even with this background I was unprepared for what unfolded next.

When Lynnette started the Dru Yoga teacher training course she arrived in a wheelchair. She was able to stand, shakily, for just a few of the flowing movements we taught that module. The rest she visualised.

She arrived at the second module looking considerably improved, participating in many of the movements we taught over those four days.

Six months later, at the start of the course's third module, Lynnette walked into the room, her wheelchair outside, a mute trophy to her determined yoga practice.

Just under a year later she arrived for the yoga course's fourth module with only her sticks for support. 'Where's your wheelchair?' we asked. 'Oh,' she replied in her characteristically understated way, 'I didn't think I'd need it any more so I've given it back.' That night she walked two kilometres through the city back to her accommodation.

During this time we had little knowledge of how Lynnette was achieving these remarkable outcomes. 'Well, I just did what you were teaching,' she'd say, 'visualising the techniques when I couldn't physically do them.'

We guessed there was more to it. And there was. This book is the story of how she really managed a 'miracle' – and many more triumphs of transformation to follow.

Yet perhaps Lynnette's greatest miracle is that in *A Journey to Peace Through Yoga* she makes it possible for each of us to follow in her footsteps, even if we have to start with wheels.

Andrew Wells,
Co-director, Dru Australia

How to use this book

A Journey to Peace Through Yoga has two main components, the narrative of my journey through and beyond the trials and tribulations of my life, and the practices that have enabled this journey towards wellness.

Each practice has had its place in my management of MS, for different reasons. I am not trying to write a text book on Dru Yoga and Meditation, so it is the reason itself I describe rather than the details of the practice.

I have integrated my practice into my life and experienced profound transformation as a consequence, so I have referred to practices within the story and included them at the end of each chapter to give you the opportunity to also experience this integration.

If only I could live in this space …

Most of us have experienced moments of connected-ness to our higher spiritual self; moments of sublime joy, when time seems to stop and we realise we are part of something much bigger than ourselves, when boundaries separating us from 'other' dissolve.

My earliest memories of such experiences were me rowing a dinghy by myself on Sydney Harbour, sitting on the deck of my father's boat in the stillness of a starry night and standing on the end of the boat club wharf with my face toward a howling southerly blowing across the water from Five Dock.

I had no idea why I wanted to row for hours every weekend or stand in the freezing wind with just a t-shirt, no language to express the sense of wholeness and belonging; I just knew the peace and stillness I felt was right.

Then, when a little older, after a day's walking through the Royal National Park south of Sydney, standing on the rocks with a friend, with the twinkling canopy of stars above us, looking out to sea – a feeling of sublime joy washed over us both, absolute connect-edness, even to the rocks beneath our feet.

The first time my son suckled; the first 'I know you' look exchanged between my first daughter and I; and a moment of deep connection in pregnancy with my youngest.

All these moments and more speak of a sense of continuum – recognition of one life-force that runs through us all. Perhaps even a sense of coming home in some indefinable way.

The first time I recognised this in a spiritual context was during a meditation workshop with a Zen master, in Byron Bay – where else?! At the time I was feeling lost, as I had done for most of my life. I was not a spiritual or religious person. In fact, I strongly felt that the faith gene was not in my DNA! The master had come to speak at my yoga school in Bellingen and I felt incredibly drawn to him and the retreat. These days I would describe it as a "kching!" moment but back then it was just weird and compulsive.

At some point on the second day of the retreat, during my one-on-one with the master a great stillness came into the room and the space between us became illuminated; we seemed to become one and in doing so transcended each other as individuals. The only way I can describe the feeling is of coming home, in my heart.

I walked away from the retreat no longer an asthmatic.

Then later still, four years ago, alone in a hospital bed in Britain, unable to lift my head, arms or legs, in agonising pain with waves of pins and needles, tingling, numbness, and hot and cold sweeping through my body, a peace beyond description descended as I surrendered to whatever was happening to my body.

All resistance to my situation faded, and I lay in stillness, feeling my breath and simply being. A minute before I had been feeling a loneliness and despair too deep to describe in words. Then suddenly, surrender, serenity, joy and peace … home again.

If only I could live in this space. In that moment I had some sense that it wouldn't matter what the physical circumstances of my life were, I could accept this condition, whatever it was, if I could live in this space.

This was the official beginning of my journey with multiple sclerosis (MS), although, as many MS patients will tell you there are months, sometimes years of bizarre and idiosyncratic symptoms before an event big enough to go down the diagnosis route.

So, when two years later I sat in my wheelchair at a Dru Meditation weekend, unable at times to lift a glass to my mouth and still in pain, yet feeling that same peace and stillness, that same sense of surrender, I realised it was time to learn how to live in that space; and, more importantly, how to share this stillness with other disabled folk or anyone else who would listen.

What I have realised since is that this is our natural state, and that we all have the desire and the capacity to be in this state.

This is the story of my journey home, a spark of the splendour that is possible.

Intro

UP TO 2003

I have just read a testimonial from a man who has been living with terminal cancer for several years and was reminded of the millions of families in the same predicament all over the world. Last night I heard a story of a father in a re-education camp in south-east Asia and was reminded of the millions of displaced people and fractured families around the world.

In the context of these and many other stories of people surviving hardship, mine seems insignificant. There are hundreds of thousands of stories of people transcending difficulty with faith or diet or exercise regime or just by surviving, so why add another?

Simple – the more stories there are about people who have empowered themselves, and the more there are for people to read and become inspired by, the more chance there is that when we inevitably stumble into a dark period of our lives we can read about others who encountered difficulty and triumphed.

When there is only one story it can easily be passed over as the result of coincidence or an extraordinary person or wealth. The more stories we hear, and possibilities and methods we learn of, the better because somewhere in that huge pile of possibilities there might be one that inspires. If someone else can do it there's even more of a chance I can – they can't all be extraordinary. And let me tell you, I know I am not!

When Brandon Bays was diagnosed with an abdominal tumour, she already knew of people who had "cured themselves". She knew that if they could do it, so could she, and she did. Out of her healing journey came *The Journey* program, which has since helped thousands of people, including me.

In the hope that my story will help people already struggling with difficulty or provide people with the knowledge that it's possible, I want to share.

My journey is both one of healing and spirituality. I have not done this alone and now walk every step with the presence of spirit. To begin the healing journey I must first explain the rest. To understand the significance of where I am now you must first understand where I have come from.

To know where to begin is difficult because, like most stories there is no real beginning or end; it is more like a continuum of experiences from conception (and even here there are ancestors and the possibility of past lives) to the last breath. Even with MS there was a period when little symptoms appeared before the big ones bit.

My life until 2003 had never been exactly easy or even particularly happy. I was born the fifth child in a family in crisis – mental illness, financial stress and anger, lots of anger.

Through my childhood I felt like the runt of the litter: asthma, bronchitis, near-fatal tick poisoning, back pain and intense menstrual pain. At twenty I was diagnosed with poly-cystic ovaries and endometriosis.

I grew up feeling bullied by everyone and everything, including a sexual assault that I hid from everyone, even myself. Emotionally isolated, I shrank from reality into my fantasies.

I didn't expect anyone to really like me and I think I didn't expect to really like anyone else, despite desperately wanting to. I saw the world and everything as something to be feared.

Yet running through this, like an underground fresh water stream, was an empathy and compassion for the suffering others. I felt unable to properly compete in the material world because it would inevitably result in someone else or me losing, but my insecurities prevented me from fully embracing this extraordinary gift of compassion – I couldn't possibly be that big, I couldn't take the risk. There existed a hidden fear that if I stuck my head up it would get cut off.

So, rather than becoming a light of compassion, I became resentful of the 'Suns' of the world – the leaders and the stars. Why wasn't I getting that recognition? Why couldn't I shine? I now know it was because I wasn't expressing my gift, and didn't even know that what I had was a gift; to me it felt like a burden. I felt like a loser in the material, successful world, and that feeling expressed itself as resentment in every aspect of my life.

My intimate relationships were dysfunctional and my friendships always seemed spasmodic at best, one sided at worst.

Professionally, I had no direction. I wanted success but couldn't manifest it, and seemed to sabotage my opportunities.

As I look back I see a life lived on the edge of emotional meltdown: occasionally dipping into depression, occasionally being targeted by people I called "do-gooders", but mostly managing at least a semblance of control. My friends at university would exclaim at how calm I seemed but they didn't see the seething mass of insecurity the calm exterior masked. I envied their ability to express themselves, to be themselves.

I just felt numb to the rest of the world.

Yet even still, there always seemed to be a guardian angel stepping in when life got too tough or too close to disaster. No single incident was extreme, and I did manage to keep life afloat, with my children being the shining lights of my life. I found a happiness in loving my children I had not found in any other aspect of my life.

So, when the calendar year turned from 2002 into 2003, I thought my life was on the way up. I was happily pregnant with my third child, we had bought an amazing block of land that was going to be our place in the sun and I was planning to teach casually to make ends meet, as well as writing chapters in a maths text.

Boy was I wrong!

The next eighteen months were to be my *annus horribilus* … and a half!

My Annus Horribilus...
and a Half

JANUARY – MARCH 2003

First to hit was a dearth of casual teaching, moving our already stretched finances toward insolvency.

Then, an inexplicable fatigue followed. Not just the usual tiredness that can come with pregnancy but rather an extreme fatigue, from the moment I woke up until the moment I went to sleep. I felt so heavy and could easily fall asleep at any time of the day; sometimes I could hardly lift my arms and legs.

I was unable to think creatively or logically, in fact I was often unable to think at all! With this came a depression and emotional numbness, a kind of withdrawal and mental fogginess preventing me from meeting my writing, caring or any other commitments. I knew I was letting everyone down but couldn't do anything about it.

Our finances in crisis, we moved onto our land in a caravan and the old Lange family 18 foot square canvas

1

tent. Our 'house' belongings went into the tent and two children, husband and pregnant wife moved into a small caravan and annex in autumn on the Southern tablelands – and it was cold! With no bathroom, we made a nuisance of ourselves at our new neighbours' houses, subsisting on a caravan stove and fridge, and a 'deep-drop' hole in the ground as our dunny – life was very basic!

If one could let go of being cold, broke and very, very tired (not to mention slightly mad) for a moment or two, there was breathtaking beauty in the simplicity of this life.

The ice crystals that formed on the *inside* of the annex roof where Matthew (my husband) and I slept transformed our humble abode into a magical palace so that each morning I woke feeling like a fairy queen. The landscape outside was similarly transformed into a magical garden as the sun reflected off the frosty glass and frozen puddles. All surfaces seemed to glint, surrounding us in endless rainbow sparkles.

At night after the children went to bed, underneath velvety sky scattered with more stars than I thought possible, Matthew and I sat around the open fire. For the first time in my life I became aware of the phases of the jewel of the night sky, the moon, the beginning of a love affair with Chandra (Sanskrit for moon) that continues to this day.

It felt like an adventure and I felt intrepid and still feel a pull toward the simplicity of that time … with the inclusions of a bathroom … and maybe some thermals.

But it was about to change ...

May – June 2003

A trip to Sydney for Mother's Day in early May was to have quite dramatic consequences. The weekend with my family was lovely but on the Sunday evening before leaving for the three hour drive home, I started to feel contractions. The baby wasn't due until July.

An ultrasound revealed a low placenta, and low level contractions were recorded. A history of life-threatening post-partum bleeds was considered, as was the fact that our land was over an hour's drive from the nearest neo-natal unit, and it was strongly suggested I stay in Sydney.

To add a little spice to the mix, our second car had been stolen from outside my sister's house while I was in hospital. Fortunately it was found within 24 hours with minimal damage.

The wrench from my children was almost unbearable – for them and me. The pressure on our family unit was intense; Matthew brought the children to Sydney as often as possible, while being a single parent, fending off creditors and trying to hold down a job.

I was tired and increasingly disengaged. An experienced alternative therapist said my body was just too tired to stay pregnant and that was exactly how I felt. I think I slept for six weeks and could have slept for six more. I was supposed to be writing chapters in maths texts but found it so difficult to concentrate for any length of time.

June – July 2003

I finally returned home on a Sunday in mid-June. Matthew had found a larger caravan with a potbelly stove which would give us more room (and warmth) when the baby came, so once again I was feeling optimistic. Four days later my waters broke, and in the early hours of Thursday morning we made a very quick drive to Canberra. Nicola Carriadd was born after an induced but straightforward four-hour labour, the following day.

The older children fell in love with their younger sister minutes after she was born. Celebration and relief followed. We had a healthy baby, the placenta was delivered in one piece and there was no post-partum haemorrhaging (I have a history of retained placentas and life threatening post-partum haemorrhaging).

Once again I felt that intense rush of love as my new child was placed in my arms and she suckled at my breast for the first time. Bliss! We had done it!

That night or the next I experienced the strangest sensation. Each time I laid down I had the nauseating feeling of falling backwards into space and my lungs felt like they were too heavy to fill. I thought the lung thing was just a stress-related return of asthma, although I must admit, asthma had never felt like that – I couldn't expand my chest, it felt so heavy.

The midwife gave me a Ventolin, even though my oxygen levels were fine, but with no relief I sat in a chair and tried to sleep.

Even when I write this now, with the benefit of

hindsight and the knowledge of where these symptoms were leading, it sounds bizarre, but trying to explain it to overworked midwives who are thinking about babies and the next delivery and ensuring that all scores were met, it must have seemed quite ridiculous and probably psychological.

Day three, Nicola and I were sent home. A healthy baby and a mum who knew which end to put a nappy on and which end to put a breast in could go home, vacating a bed in an overcrowded system.

We moved into the new caravan to set about getting to know my baby and reuniting with my two big children. I was still falling back into space but I was so happy to be home, so happy to be breastfeeding again, so happy to be with my children.

This was about to change.

A check with my local doctor two days later revealed a baby who was indeed feeding well and putting on weight but a mother who was barely standing up. My balance was completely disrupted and I was clearly exhausted, still. Perhaps an inner ear infection, thought the doctor.

Out of fear I might fall over with the baby, the doctor wanted to admit me to hospital. Of course, the local hospital didn't have any cradles, so I would have to go to either Goulburn or Canberra Hospital.

I rang my husband and dissolved into tears to the point of being unable to speak. Now I was considered a post-natal depression risk as well. They kept Nicola and I at the doctor's surgery until Matthew arrived from work, when he convinced them to leave us in his care and took yet more time off work.

I slowly recovered from the birth and my balance improved but didn't return to the surefootedness I had grown up with, and the fatigue never really left. My doctor's concern was never voiced, although he did allude to the possibility of something more serious. "Let's hope it goes away or we will have to do some further investigations." Needless to say, I didn't go back for 'further investigations'.

Our house in Goulburn sold, at least relieving the pressure of our financial mess when the sale finalised.

July – August 2003

A few weeks after Nicola's birth, a mid-morning phone call changed our lives yet again. Matthew's mother had passed away in Wales the previous night. We managed to get enough money together for a return ticket to the UK for Matthew (knowing we could repay the money when the house settled), and neighbours we hardly knew offered the children and me a place to stay.

The moment after the farewell, as I watched him walk through the departure gates, I had a gut feeling that I was saying goodbye to him; goodbye to our relationship. As he disappeared into customs a stone sunk in my belly – he was gone.

Two weeks later he returned and my life fell apart. I was right, I had said goodbye to our relationship or at least our relationship as I had known it for the previous ten years.

As our relationship and our lives went into meltdown, tiredness and other symptoms were easily discounted as stress and due to a newborn baby feeding on demand.

And one of the first things I did was roll a cigarette. I had smoked as young adult and socially smoked for a couple of years when the children were a little older but I remember the moment I consciously lit that cigarette as an antidepressant. It was a short-term thing I thought, just to get me through this period. I managed to keep it to around ten 'racehorse' cigarettes a day but it would take almost two years to 'get me through this period' and stop, hopefully, for the last time.

With no houses to rent in our village or in the nearest town, still staying with my three children in the spare room of some very generous people who were now getting to know us very quickly, I felt homeless, destitute and devastated, like a refugee without a war.

Yet even during that time of darkness there were moments of light and moments of joy; moments when I was able to stand aside from my pain and see the best and the beautiful.

In the early hours of the morning, a few days after Matthew returned, I was writing him a letter when I felt golden effervescence rise through my abdomen and into my heart, from where it spread throughout the rest of my body. That feeling was love and I knew then that if I could live in that love it would be fine. I would be fine.

I saw rainbows in the sky, light in extraordinary

landscape, and love, in my children and yes, even in my husband.

After a few weeks of unsuccessfully looking for houses to rent, the children and I moved into a rented caravan about thirty feet away from the previous encampment on our land, where Matthew was living. I encouraged the children to approach this as yet another adventure.

We entered into a surreal period of our lives. The children were still going to school every day, Matthew was going to work every day and I was mothering my new baby.

At night after the older two children went to sleep, I would take Nicola over to our old caravan where she slept, while Matthew and I would talk into the early hours of the morning. Night after night we dissected our previous life, our past lives, ourselves and our future.

It was the strangest thing – exhausting, exhilarating, deeply painful, liberating and alive. We had never communicated with more intimacy or honesty. I was alive and in the moment; my energy waned only when I thought about what would happen or when other people asked me what would happen.

This too would change…

September 2003

The day of my 38th birthday, 15th September 2003, came and went; the children bought beautiful presents and Matthew took me to the beach for picnic. It was beautiful but something crucial was missing, even though we were both trying terribly hard to ignore it and trying terribly hard to make it right.

The 16th of September began ominously; as my husband left for work, I felt exhausted and was overcome with deep sadness. I put Nicola to sleep in the old caravan, as was our routine, and went over to the rented caravan to wash breakfast dishes. But Nicola wasn't settling for her morning sleep that day and after several attempts I brought her over to the rented caravan.

Emotional exhaustion and deep melancholy swept over my body and mind, I was over it, ready to let go – I couldn't fight anymore. I sat down on the steps of the rented caravan, allowing the thought to take hold in my mind, "I can't do this anymore".

I looked over to the old caravan with a feeling of sad nostalgia, but instead of the usual peaceful scene, plumes of black smoke were billowing from the door. A sense of panic rose through my body and leaving Nicola in the rented caravan, I ran over ... too hot and too toxic to get close. PANIC ... FEAR ... NICOLA ... AWAY

Perhaps I could have rescued stuff, perhaps I could have done more but all I could think of was getting Nicola away. We drove to the same neighbours, who by now were probably thinking we were disaster personified, and phoned the fire brigade and Matthew, then returned to wait for the firemen to arrive.

By the time I arrived back at the site, the two caravans and the tent were alight, burning beyond redemption. I stood, holding my three-month-old baby, watching every material possession and memento (even the previous day's birthday presents) from mine, my husband's and our children's lives go up in smoke.

There are no words to describe the devastation I felt in these moments. My mind retreated further into shock.

The days that followed are a blur of pain and loss and wailing children, as we all remembered things we had lost. There were very few moments I didn't hold Nicola close to my breast and thank god she hadn't settled that day or when I didn't hold the other children and thank god they had been at school.

Yet even in this week there were golden moments: a woman at the local general store who paid for our replacement underwear out of her own salary; an offer from Matthew's employers to rent us a house in Goulburn for minimal rent; and when I walked into that house and found it furnished from the garages and sheds of council employees, all I could do was cry.

Over the coming weeks there was rarely a day when we didn't arrive home to a new bag of stuff dropped by someone who had heard of our plight.

The kindness and generosity we received was uplifting but it didn't stop our hearts from slowly closing. We had a house but had lost our home and felt rootless. And after having the wind blowing between us in the caravans, my husband and I were now back in the sardine can of one roof – squeezing the intimacy out and forcing us into 'push me/pull you' territory ... still, at least it was a house and not a shanty in a refugee camp.

October – December 2003

After nearly eleven years of devoted motherhood, I began to withdraw. I felt so tired. I continued to breast-feed on demand but my focus turned inward. I missed commitments for the children, allowed bad habits to develop and was unable to dispel anger – theirs or mine. I knew I wasn't present for them and felt guilty, but I was empty, numb, and I had nothing left.

If any of my three children ever have doubts about my ability to be there for them in moments of crisis, the seeds were sown during 2003.

And in the background was the lurking suspicion, a voice telling me that all was not well in my body. "Yes, I am breastfeeding and tired and stressed ... but ... tingling, balance, weird vision, numbness at the back of my neck, sudden moments of weakness and funny little twitches on my upper lip ... strange sensations ... no, it's fine."

December 2003

Feeling no roots in Australia, no direction for children's schooling, and a desperate need for some change, we decided to see if I could work in the UK.

My son had been accelerated through Year 4 and at 11 years old was now finishing primary school. He wanted to go to boarding school, having grown up with Enid Blyton's descriptions of good food and even better friends, but 11 was just too young. Gracie was also a little lost, having spent two years in an independent school recovering from being bullied.

In addition, I needed a break from being the full-time carer. I was so empty and Matthew was happy to parent for a while.

Two weeks later I accepted a job in an inner-city school in Bristol and we were planning a move to the UK.

Then an article in a doctor's surgery about a woman's journey with MS tinkled alarm bells in my mind. Her symptoms sounded just like all the things I was experiencing.

"No, that's not me, besides the doctor is giving me a full medical and I'm fine."

There it stayed in the back of my subconscious … "new baby, fatigue, seesawing relationship, angry unsettled children, guilt over crap parenting, still feeling homelessness and moving countries. I am tired, no wonder I feel stressed, perhaps that's what's causing the symptoms?"

January 2004

Numb!

Britain in winter – cold, wet and dark.

No house to rent, moving from one motel to another.

I started teaching with our suitcases in the back of our car, not knowing where we would be sleeping each night.

Leaving Nicola for the first time was horrible– the

pain almost physical. Thank god Matthew was looking after her, regardless of the relationship between us; I knew I could trust him with Nicola. I was still breast-feeding at night.

Luckily my guardian angel prevailed and the head teacher offered me accommodation – a temporary reprieve.

In the first week, two students threatened to jump out of the second floor window, one student pole danced through a Year 10 maths class and a Year 7 student threatened me with getting his family to wait outside the school and "bash the **** out of me after school".

I was in shock, like a rabbit caught in headlights, and all I could do was live in each moment.

Yet the beauty of Wales in winter when we visited my brother-in-law was breathtaking; snow on the Brecon Beacons, green grass and moistness.

After two weeks of living and working out of a suitcase, we finally move into a house and the two children started at the local school, a lovely small village school where maybe they could breathe again … and maybe, so could I.

February 2004

We slid into a routine of sorts. I travelled into Bristol daily with my head teacher. My two older children settled into their new school and Nicola settled into her new life with daddy. The last thing I did before I left home and the first thing I did when I came home was breastfeed, and then every couple of hours in between. And Matthew cooked every night ... so nice to get home and smell dinner. Faggots in gravy – yummm!

Then, in the middle of the grind it snowed – it was so beautiful. We all took the day off to go tobogganing in Cheddar gorge, visit the sweet shop and drink hot chocolate in the snow. Cold and soggy and muddy is so much more romantic with a cup of hot chocolate in the snow on the other side of the world!

I walked up the hill to feel the cold wind on my face. I love to be on my own, facing into the wind. I felt so free ... until Nicola on my back complained and I descended ... but just for that moment I believed with my whole being that anything was possible.

With all the maturity of my adulthood and modernity of the twenty-first century in these towns, it was still a little like walking through a story book for me; there is a child-like innocence in this state of mind that soothed my pain. Maybe I could have 'happy-ever-after', after all.

It was these moments of beauty and love that prevented me from sliding into the darkness that seemed to threaten at every turn. I seemed to just manage to hold it at bay while I experienced these brief moments of joy. They were like rays of sunshine through the clouds.

And the physical symptoms were still there, becoming more pronounced; more moments of weakness, losing my balance a bit more, vision funnier and digestion getting worse. Hardly a day went by when I didn't

notice some little symptom appearing or incremen-
tally degenerating. "Just tired, just stressed."

March 2004

As February became March, the weather began to
brighten and the change in the people around me
was palpable. I thought the mood and season connection was a myth created by conspiracy theorists, but
it's real.

The staffroom in February was dark, gloomy and
downright depressing. Teachers are rarely a happy
bunch but this was ridiculous – people quite literally
just didn't smile. Not only did they not smile, they
whinged and complained, with one colleague often
sharing the statistic that teachers have the shortest life-
span after retirement – jolly.

Then the days started to get longer, the temperature warmed, the winds eased slightly and maybe, just
maybe, there was a bit more sunlight. The margins
were small but enough to lighten spirits, enough to
give people some hope of the coming spring.

Teaching also became easier, found its own rhythm.
The school was under review and the maths department under even tighter scrutiny, with the added difficulty of two non-permanent staff. So the pressure
was on to lift our professional standards and have us all
looking like perfect teachers by the end of April.

It was a little like polishing the surface so the
scum underneath doesn't show; the Barbie school
– it all looks good but if you look closely enough for

long enough you will soon realise the proportions are all wrong.

Yet my teaching practices were enhanced and my classes did actually improve. I taught all low-ability classes and two special needs, but the classes were becoming more structured and I think some of the students were actually learning something.

However, the lives of these kids were so worrying and I wondered if what I did made any difference at all. All it took was for one kid to go off and the class was lost. Tables still got thrown occasionally and kids still turned up to class stoned; the language was appalling and I still got asked if I enjoyed oral sex; fourteen-year-old girls were proud of themselves for only having nine sexual partners and boasted about 'bare-back riding'; and both boys and girls boasted about binge drug taking, while boys talked about crime they were going to commit, had already committed or knew had been committed.

Every night I came home to my little family and prayed it would not be them in a few years. They seemed so perfect, so innocent.

The strain at home was palpable. Matthew and I were not fighting; we were too numb to be fighting. There was just no joy, almost no communication.

By the end of March my physical symptoms had become so pronounced I saw my local doctor. The fear I had been suppressing was coming to the surface. The doctor began the process of referral to a neurologist and sent me to have a special eye examination.

Another appointment was made to get the results of the eye test.

April, 2004

Holidays, yeah!!!

My husband had arranged a week in Cornwall. We were all so excited. We visited Tintagel and the Eden Project in Cornwall and roamed through castles along the south coast of England but all the time I had a black cloud shading my mind. The tingles and numbness were present constantly, and the weakness and fatigue set in without a moment's notice. I forced myself through walks, up and down steps to enjoy this holiday.

"I will enjoy this holiday", was my mantra, despite feeling it was our last in innocence.

The south of England is beautiful and there were many moments to savour but the next week I had a physical crash and the visit to the doctor revealed some vision loss and a warning to my husband: "if it gets any worse, take her straight to the hospital".

The following week we returned to school and the final inspection. We passed (both the maths department and the school)! A celebratory dinner at the head's house felt remarkably uncomfortable and morose for a group of colleagues that had just passed the Barbie test. I felt detached, like only part of me was there – the part that was drinking too much and trying to be jolly and remembering that one of my colleagues really didn't smoke.

May, 2004

On the Sunday after, Matthew and I planned visits to relatives in Wales but a bath completely wiped me out and I couldn't even get out by myself. However, brief sleep and we were on our way, a little late but on our way. We took a beautiful walk through the Welsh countryside but I felt so weak and exhausted I only just got back.

"Be careful, don't overdo it. Look after yourself."

"I'll be fine. Stop fussing."

… Famous last words.

Monday morning and my lift forgot to pick me up. I knew I couldn't drive the 40 minutes to Bristol so I called in sick. By mid-morning I couldn't sit up without leaning over to one side; by lunchtime, I couldn't stand or walk, and the by the afternoon I couldn't sit up at all.

My husband took me to the local hospital and I was admitted immediately. The nightmare had begun.

Another wrench from my children, more pressure on my husband – I can see him in shock as he seemed to shut down a little more in each moment. Nicola changed her routine again, breastfeeding through the day when Matthew brought her into the hospital, and bottles at night. She was nearly twelve months old and the first night she cried inconsolably; all Matthew could do was hold her. Gabriel, at 11, couldn't bear to come into the hospital and Grace at nine came because she couldn't bear not to, in fear I was dying.

The pain is my family's eyes made anything I

felt in my body seem inconsequential. I had always soothed them when they felt pain, I had always been there for them, had always nurtured them; it had been my job. Now, I had nothing to give them. I couldn't even tell them I wasn't dying because I didn't know myself. I felt like I was failing them. Another layer of my identity as mother was being ripped away from me, again.

Within 24 hours I had been given two lumbar punctures, X-rays and a CT scan of my brain. The lumbar punctures returned positive for protein in the spinal fluid so I was booked in for a full body MRI.

Come Saturday night, I had been in hospital since Monday and was again in excruciating pain. Matthew had long gone home with Nicola and Grace, and I felt incredibly alone.

I couldn't lift my head off the pillow without intense searing pain, nausea and dizziness; wave after wave of seemingly random neurological sensations were sweeping through my body – pins and needles, numbness, heat, cold and tingles. Feeling panic and fear rising, I struggled against this state; against the fire-works going off in my brain.

Then for some reason I started to breathe more deeply and lie very still. I surrendered. I felt so small lying in the bed, so I found the centre and slipped into the silence amid the noise. Time stopped. Life came from somewhere deep inside of me and this is where I stayed, in this very deep place. The pain swirled around me and I sat in the stillness allowing it to move further from my awareness. There was a feeling of deep peace, perhaps even joy.

Is this meditation?

I moved deeper, into an image of my husband as a teddy bear being ripped apart, with me pulling on one side. I had to stop pulling if he is to stay in one piece. I let go and in that moment pledged to love him unconditionally, regardless of his love or not for me, whether we stayed together or not, till his last breath ...

After this night, it started. I 'meditated' in bed as much as I could. I didn't really know what to do; I just sat in stillness and breathed, allowed the stillness in my breath to become peace in my mind. Peace in the context of turmoil. Meditation became my safe place and I had a feeling if I stayed in this safe place, my physical condition would become inconsequential.

On Monday, it was time for my MRI. The transport driver was expecting me to be ambulant and I could barely stand. I was claustrophobic and as I lay down on the MRI bed with the machine behind me, fear started to rise.

The ear plugs went in and the cage came down over my face, more fear, almost panic ... and then I remembered to breathe. I closed my eyes and breathed into my belly and the fear began to recede. I surrendered again, the bed slid back into the tunnel and the scan began.

It was so loud. Any feelings of claustrophobia are exacerbated by the constant rhythmical noise in different pitches and volumes. I consciously relaxed my body; first my toes, then my feet, my legs, my abdomen, chest, hands, arms, back, neck and head. For nearly two hours they scanned my head and spine, and afterwards I felt surprisingly relaxed and calm, although utterly exhausted.

The scan showed inflammation in my brain and the possibility of a clot so I had to return for another scan and take anti-coagulants in the meantime.

Tuesday brought my first physiotherapy session. I tried so hard but I didn't know where my legs were. I used to have core stability but then I collapsed from the core; I fell twice because I was trying so hard. I cried in frustration but inwardly I was screaming.

"AHHHHHHH!!!"

When I returned to my bed the staff arranged a walking frame for me. A WALKING FRAME?! "But I don't need a walking frame, I'm not even forty", my mind screamed. "What's happening to me?"

Then Matthew arrived with Nicola and I was reminded of love. I breastfed and cuddled and smiled, and Matthew fed me. Thank god for Matthew, thank god for Nicola.

After they left I tried sitting. Plumped up by cushions I sat, closed my eyes and breathed. A feeling of calm descended once again and there I sat all afternoon. Surrender. I used my walking frame and made it to the toilet and back – no more bed pans, yay!

I was told my meditation created a sense of calm in my ward; a very frightened patient I had been focussing on became calmer. Probably a coincidence, I thought.

Another patient told me my voice was therapeutic, calming – I wished it would work for me.

The second MRI was shorter and far less tiring, and there was no fear – I knew I could breathe through the scan. The results showed no blood clot but questionable blood vessel structure, possibly indicative of a different disease, which first sounded like a relief and then a rather hideous alternative to MS – yes, there are worse fates than MS, kind of comforting in a weird, morose, Monty Python kind of way.

I was transferred to a hospital in Bristol for another test (which is called a cerebral angiogram). The anaesthetist inserted a catheter into a blood vessel in my groin which goes all the way up into the base of my brain. He injected dye through the catheter so the vascular structure of my brain could be seen on X-ray scans.

There were horror stories of both diseases in my new ward, as well as undiagnosed neurological horror stories, so the outcome of the test didn't really matter. I felt strangely detached and calm.

How bizarre to watch the structure of my brain emerge as the dye passed through the vascular network and the cold, metallic feeling filled my awareness. The brain is really amazing, so beautiful … and I was thinking these thoughts while watching it on the screen … so weird but very, very cool!

Well, not the alternative, so I am diagnosed with probable MS. After about a month in hospital, I am discharged with a pile of reading about living with MS (I am not wearing those tracksuit pants, no matter how easy they are to put on, and those bras are sooo ugly), a walking frame for now and sticks for later, maybe.

Even with the walking frame I could walk no longer than the end of the ward without the risk of my legs collapsing beneath me and my right leg was still dragging along the ground and twisting inward, so I had to get a wheelchair (a wheelchair?! What's that about?).

I needed physiotherapy, occupational therapy, speech therapy, continence counselling, psychological counselling, MS Society, MS therapy centres, nutritional advice, cripple clothes and, and, and … my head was spinning but at least I was going home.

June 2004

I was home from hospital, trying to wrap my head around what had happened and the implications for my identity.

"Who am I now that I am disabled? I have lost my relationship, my sense of history and faith in myself, my physical possessions, my home, my self-image as a devoted mother and now my body – what is there left?"

"At least I can still teach."

Strangely, I missed my students while I was in hospital. All of my classes were coming together, I was starting to see progress – some students were actually learning and the year 9 and 11 students were preparing for their exams and some were actually trying. Students from other classes were even trying to transfer into my classes.

I felt like I had let them down; I had promised I

would stay until the end of the academic year. They had had so many teachers.

"I really need to get back."

I wasn't sure how I could manage the stairs but the management valued my teaching and were talking about extending my contract, so I thought they would find a solution, maybe find a classroom on the ground level.

"I'm sorry, we can't take you back, you are an insurance risk."

I couldn't say goodbye to my students. I wasn't even allowed to clear my desk while the students were in the school.

I put the phone down, not even able to cry. Something snapped inside my head and life became surreal; a Dada painting as I watched it float away. I became detached, a witness. I felt stripped of all identity, just a naked form. I was a house swept empty by a huge wind. The windows were banging, the doors were hanging open and there were no furnishings … nothing …

I think this moment marked the end of my *annus horribilus … and a half.* It was also the end of my life as it was … like a small death … yet as with all deaths, it was also a beginning. The beginning of my recovery. The beginning of a life so beautiful I couldn't possibly have imagined it then.

What Choice Do I Have?

JULY 2004

After the phone call of doom I went deeper into shock but the subsequent detachment was perhaps my saviour because I just got on with the life in front of me. Perhaps it was good to have lost everything because I was starting anew. I no longer had an identity to protect or hide behind, it was just me.

I thought about the things I thought I would never do again – play tennis, row, sail, climb a cliff or dance all night – and cried, then felt grateful that I had at least had the opportunites to do them at all. I thought about things I would never do at all and cried, then thought maybe I wouldn't have done them at all, anyway.

My brother joked now I could go to the disabled Olympics (which was as close as I would ever get to an Olympic event), and finally get a car-park in Sydney; I laughed.

I went to the local MS centre, and when the

counsellor realised how recently I had been diagnosed she was shocked by how quickly I had come.

"What choice do I have? I can hardly deny that I am sitting in a wheelchair or using a walking frame."

Later I had to stop going because it became too confronting but when I was first diagnosed it was a lifeline of information and reality – there is so much information about MS but there is nothing more 'real' than talking to other people with the illness. We spend so much time thinking our symptoms are weird and that we are imagining them, it is invaluable to exchange stories with other folk who are in the same position.

So began the rounds of therapists and social workers. Not a week went by without at least one health professional or social security personnel gracing our doorstep, and each time I retold the same story and described the same symptoms. And each time they nod sympathetically and gave me more exercises or more forms or both. I felt like I was drowning in information and Velcro (an in-joke for disabled readers).

"Do I have to do this again and again and again?"

Yes I do, and I have to smile and imagine each person is the first person I've told it to because it's not their fault there have been multitudes before them. Each form has to be filled out with worse case scenarios, and of course each time reminded me what the worse case scenarios were and frequently brought them on.

And social security in Britain – demeaning, dehumanising, depressing and de-anything-that's good!

I don't know what the best practice might be but I do know this isn't it.

Much of the time I was serene and accepting, but occassionally an indescribable rage would take hold and, "I want to go to Glastonbury and punch a hippy, especially that one with the funny hat" (from a previous family trip to Glastonbury). It became a running joke; a way of diffusing the frustration. And no, I didn't ever go to Glastonbury and punch a hippy, even the one with the funny hat!

I did however read the *Little Book of Happiness* and the *Little Book of Compassion* by the Dalai Lama; and an autobiography by his sister. I learnt the mantra of compassion and began to silently chant it in my mind as often as I could remember (see **Practice of Compassion** *pg. 27*). There was something so soothing about the concepts of acceptance and compassion; something inexplicably soothing about the six syllables I was repeating over and over again.

"Om mani padme hum."

The practice of compassion

In the Dalai Lama's Little Book of Happiness, he says there is always someone who is worse off than you, so when we are feeling unhappy because of our circumstances, imagine this person/s and how they might feel.

This is the different perspective I was talking about when you hear other people's stories.

This has become a practice for me. I imagine

people who are suffering the same difficulties I am, but worse, and in my mind I send them what it is I need.

Invariably I find someone soon after doing this little meditation and give them a massage or hug or do some other random act of kindness.

Believe it or not it works. This practice never ceases to lighten my load, while reducing my need for what I have just given to someone else and giving out, all at the same time.

And if the urge arises, chant:

"Om mani padme hum."

What is MS?

MS is thought to be an auto immune disease. That means that something goes wrong with the immune system and it begins attacking an aspect of self; in the case of MS, the central nervous system (CNS)

Multiple Sclerosis means many scars, referring to the multiple sites of inflammation on myelin sheaths throughout the CNS in a person with MS. The myelin sheaths are a fatty layer around the nerve fibres. Their role is twofold: to provide protection for the fibre (think insulation) and improve conductivity of nerve impulses along the nerve fibre (think catalyst).

Disease occurs when the immune system attacks the myelin sheaths, creating inflammation and ultimately damaging the nerve fibres themselves. In worst case scenarios, large patches of nerve tissue are permanently damaged, leaving the person with permanent and often crippling dysfunction.

Nerve fibres can re-myelinate but the repair is never as good as the original and is easily derailed, especially by heat (the reason most MS patients experience exacerbations to some degree in response to an increase in body temperature). Hence the function of repaired neurones is usually impaired, even at the best of times.

Nerve damage can occur to any part of the CNS, so any function can be impaired. Therefore, the range of MS symptoms is broad and often bizarre, particularly initially. Furthermore, MS can be progressive, episodic, episodic-progressive or in remission.

It is a degenerative disease so the majority of people with MS (and certainly the majority of people I have spoken with) experience deterioration in their condition through their lifetime. At its worst, MS results in physical dependence resulting in the need for full time care in a hospice or nursing home. This degree of deterioration can occur in any age group, from teens to the elderly, although is in the minority of MS experiences.

Alternatively, some people have one episode and never have another. Of course, when we are first diagnosed, we all want to be that person. In between are people whose symptoms are mild and relatively easy to manage, people whose symptoms vary every day through the day (that's me), and everything in between.

All states of denial, acceptance, anger, depression and management also prevail. Sometimes within the same person, sometimes within the same day!

In a nutshell, it is difficult to make generalisations about symptoms, clinical path or experiences of people with MS. In this section I will describe many MS symptoms and if I miss out on any, I apologise. Please send me a polite email or letter and I will amend it for the next edition!

Table 1: MS symptoms

BODY PART/ FUNCTION	SYMPTOMS
Neurological sensations	Tingles, pins and needles, numbness, hot and cold not related to external or internal conditions (infection or hormones)
Eyes	Blurred vision; reduced peripheral vision, colour disturbances, visual disturbances, after effects of light changes, vision loss
Mobility	Reduced mobility, loss of mobility, reduced balance, loss of balance
Arms and hands	Reduced fine motor control, weakness, pain, pins and needles, reduced sensation, tremors
Skin	Reduced sensation, numbness
Hearing	Reduced hearing due to muffling, tinnitus, reduced ability to determine volume of one's own voice
Digestion	Slow digestion, constipation, cramping, gas, gastric reflux and throat dysfunction
Cognitive	Cognitive dysfunction, memory loss, inability to concentrate, confusion, fogginess
Neck	Rigidity and pain
Pain	Pins and needles, ache, random pain, sharp pain, and pain as a side effect of other symptoms
Propioception	Reduced ability (sometimes total inability) to know where your body is in space.
Speech	Slurred speech, inability to find the right word, stutter, reduced ability to get one's tongue around the sounds of speech

Swallowing	Muscle spasm closing the throat, quick fatigue of swallowing muscles resulting in inability to swallow, loss of gag reflex
Coughing	Loss of cough reflex, fatiguing of muscles involved in coughing
Bladder	Incontinence, retention, inability to recognise fullness of bladder
Spasticity	This can affect the limbs and the torso
Feet	Spasticity, foot roll, foot drop, pins and needles
Muscles spasms	Can occur in any limb, usually legs, or face, resulting in odd tics and movements of the arms and legs
Fatigue	Waking up tired and getting worse through the day and exhaustion (extreme heaviness in every part of the body) that overwhelms you unexpectedly, resulting in the need to lie down... now
Heaviness	Extreme heaviness in any limb, all of the limbs, chest, head/neck or the whole body
Heat sensitivity	All of the symptoms listed above can be exacerbated by an increase in body temperature of as little as 2 degrees C.
Facial effects	Muscle spasms and palsy effects the muscles of the face, effecting the shape and appearance of the face
Sexual dysfunction	Erectile dysfunction, loss of sensation, inability to orgasm

This is by no means meant to be a definitive list of the symptoms but it is an indication of the impact MS can have. We can experience one or all or anything in between. They can occur in isolation or together; progressively, all the time or spontaneously without warning.

Each person's experience of MS is subjective and to really understand you need to hear their experience. So tighten your seat belts and prepare to ride the MS rollercoaster with me for the next few pages.

Again, this is not meant to be an encyclopaedia of MS and there are many people with worse experiences of MS than me, different symptoms and worse experiences of each symptom I describe; no two people will describe the same story or the same set of symptoms. I do hope if you have MS, you find something that resonates and if you don't have MS, you get a better idea of what living life with MS is like.

Pain

There are different types of pain that come with MS and we can experience one or all of them at different times, and sometimes if we are unlucky, all of them or a number at once. Again, we all have our own stories and this is my experience of the pain of MS.

For example, as I write this I have an ache through my right leg, from my thigh down through the leg into my foot. This ache comes as a prelude and accompaniment to my leg going 'off-line'. I am also feeling the same ache in my right arm, from my shoulder down into my hand.

At the same time I am feeling an ache down the centreline of my brain, at the top; it is like there is an axe blade sitting between the two hemispheres of my brain, just at the top, and every so often someone gives it a little tweak, sending a sharp almost electric pain like lightning streaking across the surface of my brain (a bit like the feeling of an acupuncture needle going into the crown). The ache is constant but the sharp pain lasts only a few seconds to remind me I'm alive.

Staying with the head for a moment, I have also experienced terrible headaches since MS. These headaches are similar to migraines in that they come with a feeling of pressure around my skull, nausea, sensitivity to light and sound, yawning and confusion. Sometimes they build up through the day and sometimes by evening I need to lie down; and sometimes they are rip-snorting by 10am. I rarely get them these days and when I do the best answer is meditation.

Also there is 'pins and needles', a neurological symptom that can be very painful. It usually occurs in the limbs but I have experienced waves of pins and needles through my whole body.

Then there is the random pain that seems to occur spontaneously and disappear spontaneously, with no apparent cause or cure (not unlike MS itself we might say). Fortunately mine have been fleeting.

Oh, and abdominal pain due to poor digestion and constipation; gas and cramping. Sometimes I would dread meals because of the pain that would undoubtedly occur afterwards and it would usually stop just in time for the next meal.

Then of course there is the pain as a side effect of the symptoms.

Muscle pain from long periods of immobility and/or posture imbalance and/or spasticity.

I have never been very comfortable sitting in any position but cross-legged, and here I was, spending hours in a wheelchair. I did try to sit well but I often felt too tired to hold my spine upright and shoulders back so I often ended up slumping while listing to one side, usually my right. My back was sore, my neck was sore and my bum was sore.

As time went on I did learn to sit cross-legged in my wheelchair, pulling my legs up onto the seat, but even that for long periods gets uncomfortable and I had to lift the arm rest to really be comfortable, which has its own difficulties.

I remember in the first two modules of the yoga teacher training, I would come in from morning tea with a pen and drink in my cup holder then forget and lift the arms of the chair up to cross my legs and everything would fall onto the floor behind me – just a little embarrassing, (did I mention there are cognitive dysfunction symptoms of MS?). Then the scurrying of my peers and helpers to pick up the flotsam was even more embarrassing. Of course now I just laugh.

There is a related pain that occurs from the base of the neck up into the base of the skull (and I have now met another MS patient who understood instant-ly what I meant). It is accompanied by rigidity in the neck (like trying to turn the steering wheel of a car with power steering, after the power has been turned off), and a feeling of pressure in my brain. "Like some-one has hit you with a four by two in the back of the neck", said my new friend.

And finally, my joints. Sometimes my joints just ache and there is very little I can do about it other than meditate. When I am hot, premenstrual, tired or symp-tomatic, my joints ache, particularly my feet. I have learnt to hold my hand over the offending joint(s) and stay there until the ache recedes. I may have to do this often through a day but it does help.

The most effective way I have found to deal with the pain is to make myself more spacious, relax at a very deep level and welcome the pain – surrender (see **Meditation for headaches** p. 58). This becomes quite a powerful meditation, enabling me to sit in the centre of the pain while it rages around me. The downside is that functioning while in this state takes lots and lots of practice.

Mobility

Mobility is compromised in MS patients for so many different reasons and we may experience all of these issues or just one or two; regardless, it is debilitating and we do deserve our disabled parking stickers, regardless of how well we look.

One reason for reduced mobility is fatigue. A person with MS may look perfectly well when they first get out of a car or walking around their house, but ask them to walk any distance (and this could even be as short as 5 metres), and we will be exhausted and dragging our feet by the end. This fatigue may not only affect our legs but every area of our functioning. When this happens we need to have a rest until the fatigue passes.

Muscle weakness is another factor in reduced mobility. The muscles in our legs are too weak to lift our feet off the ground, or we can lift them off the ground but can't make a very big step so we appear to shuffle.

When I was learning to walk after my first exacer-bation in Britain, I used to lift my hip up to get my leg off the ground. This was creating alignment problems all the way along my spine and a physiotherapist at the local MS centre encouraged me to use my walking frame instead of my sticks, so I was more protected from the risk of tripping.

It was a pride thing for me: I could walk faster and didn't feel so disabled but once again I had to sur-render and break the habit (it was already difficult to break); my back pain eased.

Once when being fitted for a foot brace to reduce tripping (due to foot roll – another problem for mobil-ity), I was quite horrified to realise the quads (front thigh muscles) were too weak to lift my right foot off the ground.

Again, I couldn't believe I wasn't lifting my foot off the ground. No wonder I was tripping so much. Even now, there are days when my right foot doesn't come off the ground very far, and that's with a lot of effort.

This explains a symptom I had felt as early as 2001. I remember walking up a slope, trying to walk quickly and feeling incredible heaviness in my thighs, not being able to lift my legs. It felt so humiliating to be that weak. I was sure I wasn't that unfit but I was having the same difficulty with stairs. I still struggle with inclines.

The muscles lifting my right foot were also weak which meant my toes were dragging on the ground, creating a constant trip hazard, as well as the tendency for my foot to turn inwards and roll when taking a step. I still have stretched muscles in my right ankle.

When I was first getting out of my wheelchair, and for a long time afterwards I really had to concentrate on putting my foot flat on the ground and maintain square alignment with my hips (still do sometimes). Every step was conscious.

And sometimes my body just stops. It might be my legs or my whole body – it just stops. Sometimes I will be able to give it a kick-start by moving my leg(s) independently (use one of my sticks or ask on of my family members to push my leg), or sometimes it just stops and there's no moving it until whatever is making it stop recovers.

I remember one occasion in Britain during my recovery when I left the lounge room to go up the stairs to bed, which was a bit of an ordeal at the best of times. I was exhausted and half way up the stairs when my whole body stopped working. It wasn't a feeling of weakness; I just couldn't make it work anymore.

I sat down for a rest and suddenly felt overwhelmed by fatigue, so I laid down. I don't think I went to sleep but I lay half way up the stairs for quite some time.

Eventually Matthew realised I was there and asked me if I needed some help.

"No, I'm OK I'm just having a rest."

"You can't stay there all night, I'll help you up."

And so he did.

This has happened many times along my journey

with MS, with both legs and arms, and one of the areas yoga and meditation has been the most helpful with.

Balance is another factor in reduced mobility. Sometimes even if all the muscles are working and pelvic floor is engaged, taking a foot off the ground to take another step can create the 'death wobble of doom'. It begins as a little over-balance to one side, followed by an over correction to the other side, and so on until I pass the point of no return and go over.

I lost my centre of balance so I didn't know where I had to get back to and even standing could induce the death wobble of doom. As a consequence, before I surrendered to walking aids I never walked very far from a wall or hand rail; even now walking can sometimes feel precarious and I still feel I need to concentrate going down stairs.

Sometimes I still use walking aides if my balance feels compromised. I no longer have any pride associated with my sticks – it is far more humbling to fall than it is to use a stick or two.

Collapsing is hard to explain and I still don't really know why it happens. At its worst it begins with core stability collapse (see *Core stability* p.59): like pulling out the foundation block in a block tower, the whole tower collapses or kind of crumbles.

At its least, one or other of my legs (more often the right) will collapse underneath me. If my balance is good this will only generate a lurch to that side (sometimes almost unnoticeable). However, combine this with loose balance and it can lead to the death wobble of doom.

Combine these symptoms with speech difficulties and manual dexterity problems, and it is no wonder people with MS often get mistaken and misjudged for drunks as we lurch precariously form one side to the other, slur our words (if we can find the right one) and fumble with our money.

I remember quite a few people who were cold and distant with me before my relapse in 2006 who then seeing me in a wheelchair after my exacerbation, suddenly became incredibly kind and helpful. It was only then I realised I had been judged as a drunk in the middle of the day with a young child. No wonder they were cold and distant.

Of course all these mobility issues carry with them the risk of falling, with the associated risks of further injury. So when I surrendered to walking aids, it not only gave me greater independence but also safety. Mind you, pride still intervened at times and I didn't use them as much as I could.

Speech

Speech difficulties are also varied and they can be permanent or episodic (for me they have been episodic). And again, they can occur simultaneously or independently of each other

Slurring like I am inebriated is one symptom I have experienced, particularly in the beginning and during the 2006 exacerbation. Getting my tongue in the right shape to form the words is another. This results in a kind of incoherent stutter, stopping and starting sentences as I try to find a way to say what I want to say.

Finally, and most embarrassingly, finding the right word. Again people say, "Oh, that's just a normal part of aging", except I was 38 when it started and it's not the usual grasping for a word, rather saying a similar sounding word or a word in the similar family of words. As soon as the word comes out I know it's wrong but until that moment I am sure it's right.

My children have many instances when I have said nonsensical things in public situations but I will tell just one that happened a few months after returning from the UK.

It was the day of Grace's birthday party and I went into town to get some last-minute party supplies. I was tired and a little dodgy but OK.

Gabe had asked for a big bottle of a new drink with a name something like 'Viage'. Around the supermarket I went ticking off my list but I could only see small bottles of drink on the shelf. So, with a full trolley of 10 year-old party food, I walked up to the man at the checkout.

"Do you have any big bottles of Viagra?"

As soon as it came out of my mouth I realised it was wrong (very wrong) but there was nothing I could do. He blushed all colours of the rainbow and choked slightly. Then, completely tongue-tied, I took him to the drink aisle to show him what I meant. On reflection, goodness knows what he thought I was going to do with him in the drinks aisle having asked for a big bottle of Viagra and he never looked at me in the same way again. In fact, he hasn't looked me in the eye since that day.

Vision

Visual difficulties are again a mixed bag, widely varying between people and within people. I know my vision issues come and go and, as with all my MS symptoms, can have rapid onset.

The first noticeable visual interference was showers of sparks in my vision. This began in 1999 and was often associated with heat (I was regularly playing tennis in Bellingen, and it was often very hot and in full sun), physical activity or showers/baths. This continues although much more sporadically than it did, and strangely, often when I am shaving my right armpit in the shower – go figure?!

Other special effects in my vision are floating paisley shapes, textured surfaces where they should be flat and more recently patches of colour, usually blue. People pay for experiences like these and I get them for free. I guess that makes me lucky.

Next came a blurring at the periphery of my vision; more on the right than the left. This also came with a physical feeling around my eyes that was often a prelude to the actual loss, often an ache similar to the ache in my legs and arms.

Then, of course, there is the blurring of the whole visual field. After a while, you forget it's abnormal until someone else mentions it as a symptom.

And finally, it takes a relatively long time for my eyes to adjust between light and dark, and I perceive after-images for quite a long time.

My visual disturbances are, however, insignificant compared to some. I have known people who have had to give up driving jobs because they couldn't focus their eyes or had permanent double vision; where reading was reduced to large print and talking books; and others who have completely lost their vision for months, only to have it return equally randomly.

Cognitive function
(or should I say, dysfunction)

This is the most difficult symptom for me to write about. It is the symptom I have dreaded the most.

I think for me there are three categories of my MS derived cognitive dysfunction: memory, concentration and analytical ability.

My memory dysfunctions include words, names, ability to rote learn facts (thank god I learnt my times tables in primary school), if I have just done something and appointments. Essentially, short term memory and the ability to learn and retain information.

I know we lose memory skills as we get older but this is different and episodic, just like my other symptoms.

My MS brain just doesn't want to be loaded with facts and figures. At first this was disastrous but maybe having a brain with more room for being present is not a bad thing (but it is nice when you can remember what you did with the ... what was I looking for?).

Concentration is linked with analytical ability because sometimes I just can't think. My mind becomes foggy and I can't even do simple calculations. Concentration, focus and even conversation becomes difficult; reading is a frustratingly word-by-word affair. Sometimes you could probably understand what I am reading by watching my lips silently form the words.

The memory difficulties are constant at a low level and sporadically more intense and the brain fog is sporadic. Nonetheless, when the two hit together, it makes managing life, juggling all the commitments around children, students and cripple appointments (doctors, therapists, case workers, social security etc) very challenging.

Taste and smell

My senses of taste and smell come and go. They are often dulled when I am pre-menstrual (along with my other symptoms), and when I am symptomatic both taste and smell are quite bland or my taste is sometimes bitter.

While a little frustrating at a gourmet meal, it was great when I first started the restricted diet because all the food tasted the same anyway, so that not eating my favourite foods didn't matter.

Again, this is not a debilitating symptom on its own but can be another symbol, a reminder, of one's physical state. It is, however, luscious when it returns;

suddenly the world tastes and smells again, almost like the first time.

Neurological sensations

It is hard to know how to classify these symptoms so I have lumped them in the same category. In essence, they are sensations that don't have an obvious physical cause and can seem relatively benign when you are not the person feeling them.

They can include pins and needles through the whole or part of the limb, patches of cold anywhere in the body (I have even experienced this in the brain, although more commonly it seems to appear in the legs e.g. backs of the thighs), patches of heat unrelated to fever or hormones, tingling in any part of the body and numbness (different to the reduced sensation in my skin).

With respect to this last sensation, it is one of the most undermining yet seemingly benign of symptoms. There have been many times through the course of MS that I have known I have a foot but not been able to feel my foot; my foot (and sometimes lower leg or hand) has been like a rubber appendage at the end of something I feel. Perceiving its existence visually and intellectually have not matched the sensation of having a foot i.e. there is a discrepancy between what we know to be true and what we are experiencing to be true.

I didn't realise how finely connected our perception of our physical reality is, and when it is disturbed in this way (or any way, probably) it undermines our physical security, our faith in our own perception of the world. This goes much deeper than just having a numb foot.

The worst experience I have had of these sensations is when I was in hospital with my very first episode in 2004. Waves of these sensations were running through my body one after the other. It was like there were fireworks going off in my brain and my body; it was out of control, going wild. There was no point of stillness except in my mind, which was where I ended up going.

Proprioception (or the lack of it)

This is another strange symptom for people with MS that undermines our faith in our own perception of our physical world.

Proprioception is our sense of knowing where our body is in the world. It is a silent sense in that when it is working well it is automatic and we don't even know we are using it. It is the sense that is highly tuned in dancers, gymnasts, athletes generally and yogis. In fact, anyone who has a high level of physical intelligence has refined proprioception, and if you are walking with reasonable coordination then yours is working just fine too.

When proprioception dysfunctions, however, that natural sense of knowing where our body parts are in relation to other body parts is disturbed. For me, this meant I would often 'forget' where my legs and arms were if I hadn't moved them for a while and would have to look to see where they were. Another strange thing that happened would be that a shadow perception in my brain where I would have the perception of where my limbs were before I moved them and where they were after, so I had to check to see which one was right.

I remember in Britain in my physiotherapy sessions doing exercises to retrain my brain to 'know' where my legs were so I could walk, and then repeating this all over again three years later.

Manual dexterity

Another term for this skill set is fine motor coordination and it basically means what we do with our hands. When your hands are working well you can write legibly (doctors and lawyers excluded), use cutlery and wrap Christmas presents. Artists, embroiderers and calligraphers have highly developed skills in this area.

When it goes wrong, any skill that requires fine motor coordination becomes difficult, if not impossible. This was far more debilitating than losing mobility because I became dependent on people for the most basic tasks: think cleaning teeth, eating, personal hygiene (a nightmare), packaging (my nemesis, sticky tape and its partner in crime, tea bags), hair and clips, buttons, shoe-laces, screwing lids, actually any kind of lids, wallets, purses, money, jewellery and drink containers – the list is endless.

When this area of my functioning is impaired at

its worst, I find it difficult to grip and use any imple-
ment that is small, and drop things all the time. This
includes cutlery, pens, sewing needles and any kitchen
tools. Again, trying to grip is like steering the power steering with the power off, and my hands ache.
Domestic skills like food preparation and washing up
are very difficult.

Occupational therapists have asked me to describe
what happens when I drop things but I don't know if
it's the strength or the coordination; I just know that
one minute I am holding something and the next
minute my hand stops working – what I was holding
is now on the floor.

Whenever my MS deteriorates my writing
becomes illegible, and I always have a limited stamina
with writing tasks so I try to keep it to writing only
what is necessary. Even now, by the end of the Samurai
Sudoku in the *Sydney Morning Herald* (five intercon-
nected Sudoku – therapy), I am the only person who
can read the numbers.

Eating is made difficult in the bad times, not just
due to the grip problem but also because it is hard to
coordinate the movements. All of my utensils need to
have larger handles and extra grips, so in my kitch-
en draws I have cripple cutlery and tools (knives and
peeler etc), and when my children set the table they
ask if I need the cripple cutlery or normal cutlery.

Word processing also has its limits – a bummer for
a writer and teacher. If I am going to write a lot I wear
wrist guards to protect my hands and keep my wrists

in a good ergonomic position, but even still I have a limited stamina so all my writing needs to be done in discrete chunks. The more I write (or if I am having a bad day) the more my typing gets very random, and my spell-check works overtime!

The low level of dysfunction I have all the time, even with recovery, includes clumsiness, messy writing, a greater than average rate of dropping things and poor fine-motor coordination.

I remember when I was first learning to make cotton wicks for the ghee lamp I use in meditation, my attempts were appalling. I rang one of my teachers in desperation and said, "Help, I'm failing Wick Making 101." My wicks are still not fabulous and will probably never look like the lovely neat wicks my teacher makes but at least they burn now and I can sit and meditate on the flame.

Eating

Eating for me was compromised not only due to the difficulties of taste and use of cutlery but also the mechanics of chewing and swallowing. When you have difficulties with muscle fatigue and coordination, it affects all the functions.

So sometimes when I eat it is difficult to get my mouth, particularly my tongue, around the coordination to chew it properly; and if it is a meal requiring a lot of chewing, I might start chewing properly and at some point my tongue and other muscles will just stop working so well. I feel 'unco' on the inside.

And the throat thing. I don't know whether this is due to my throat spasming like other muscle spasms or whether the muscles of my throat just get fatigued, but whatever the cause, the feeling is that of my throat closing and being unable swallow. This still often happens halfway through what most people call a normal size meal so it means I need to eat in small amounts, often.

At their worst, the symptoms meant I needed nutritional supplements to ensure I was getting enough nutrients. Every meal was a negotiation with my body, rather than an enjoyable repast.

Touch

Patchy reduced sensation of touch and loss of my ability to determine temperature are two of the effects to my skin. In fact, one of my first recognisable symptoms was a loss of feeling in the back of my thighs, particularly my right thigh, in 1999 in Bellingen.

I have never completely lost touch but my skin contact with the world often feels like feeling the world through a rubber glove. That means I can feel pressure but the top layers of my skin loses sensitivity. As I said, it is patchy all over my body. For some odd reason my abdomen and my forehead have been the most consistently desensitised, and still are.

Loss of touch is disconcerting and unsettling but my reduced ability to sense heat was more dangerous, both to myself and Nicola. I was banned from giving her a bath, having scalded her in water I thought was tepid, and my hands were constantly covered in scalds myself from touching water and surfaces I thought were not hot. My carers quickly learned not to ask me to test the temperature of the shower water.

Tremors

Tremors are as they sound – tremors – and they can occur, externally in the arms and the legs. My experience isn't necessarily of a resting tremor, more of a tremor in action – difficult when requiring any precision in your actions like trying to get sugar from the sugar to the cup without spilling the sugar (combine this with the odd hand-stopping-in-the-middle and this can be a risky and messy business).

Before MS I would have thought that was the end of it but now I know one can also have an internal tremor that doesn't necessarily make it to the outside and that can happen anywhere in the body. So I can feel tremors in my abdomen, thighs, arms, chest and face. The tremors don't necessarily come to the surface, so externally it looks like nothing is happening but it's all going on underneath.

The only way I have found to deal with tremors is to slow down my breathing, and hence slowing down whatever I am doing at the time, and focus on the action or the rest. This also becomes a kind of meditation so it's relaxing as well and it doesn't spill so much sugar!

Hearing

I have never been able to work out whether the hearing loss I sometimes experience is due to an interruption of the sensory process of hearing or the interpretation of what I hear but regardless, sometimes the aural world is a mumbled blur.

It is sometimes very difficult to interpret conversations or achieve clarity in terms of what people are saying. Children's language is the most difficult because children speak quickly and sometimes quietly, particularly when there is background noise like a car.

The number of times I have had to ask the people around me to repeat themselves or just let it pass by me is embarrassingly high; and in class situations I often miss crucial points in the explanation.

Digestion

I have not had an official explanation of why our digestion is affected by MS but the result is indigestion, gas, cramping pain and constipation. As an educated guess from my personal experience and bits of information from different sources, our digestive difficulties may be due to a combination of muscle fatigue and muscle coordination slowing the digestive system down, not chewing properly and a lack of activity to help digestion. Oh, and of course, stress.

The constipation in itself is due to more than one factor. One is the difficulties with digestion higher up the digestive tract, another is the muscles of the system getting tired and another seems to be the muscles spasming closed. Both the latter can create embarrassing and extremely uncomfortable circumstances, and when it first happened to me in Britain I sobbed and sobbed and sobbed with frustration, humiliation and fear.

The result is pain, bloating and gas. We often swing between the pain and discomfort of constipation to the equally painful and exhausting discomfort of diarrhoea. For those of you for whom constipation is a problem, prune juice is the ultimate bum-buster.

Muscle spasms

"It's just an excuse to give me a good kicking under the blankets," my husband used to joke about the muscles spasms that would regularly result in me kicking him in bed, although, my muscle spasming wasn't nearly as pronounced as some MS patients I have met.

I remember halfway through oxygen treatment in Britain, a fellow MS patient's leg started to spasm. Even amongst other people with MS, her embarrassment and discomfort was palpable. And it can hurt and is tiring.

Legs are a common place to experience spasms but spasming can occur anywhere in the body; sometimes a small twitch in the face, sometimes the whole body and everything in between. Spasms are spontaneous, uncontrolled and random contractions of muscle that can be both embarrassing and painful, and can result in accidents with other people or belongings.

I have experienced whole body spasming (think Peter Garrett on speed), spasming of my arms and, obviously, my legs. But you know it's the little things that make the difference and my most annoying ongoing spasm has been a little twitch in my upper lip when I am nervous, particularly during intense one-on-ones.

For example, sitting in mentoring session with my

yoga teacher and feeling intensely aware of the twitch in my right, upper lip. He probably didn't notice but to me it felt like a huge boil on the end of my nose.

I have found the only way of dealing with spasms is to stop and breathe, concentrate on the stillness within and eventually stillness forms without.

Heat sensitivity

Heat sensitivity, along with fatigue is perhaps the most universal MS symptom but really it is an exacerbation of patients' other symptoms. It is apparently due to the re-myelination process in the CNS.

When de-myelination occurs in the CNS, the body repairs the myelin around the nerve axons in a process called re-myelination. However,the repair is inexact (think putty as opposed to plaster) and when the temperature of the body increases, sometimes just by a couple of degrees, the repair loosens and the associated symptoms are exacerbated.

Heat sensitivity is such a well known aspect of MS that the MS society sponsors MS patients to get air conditioners installed in their houses. Various cooling devices are also advertised in MS publications and many words have been exchanged on networking sites to reduce the impact of heat on our lives.

The heat is not just the external temperature of the day, but also internal heat changes such as fevers, hormonal changes and food stimulations, as well as the effect of hot showers. I have been rendered completely dysfunctional by a hot shower or bath, not even being able to lift my head, let alone dress myself. Likewise with fevers and hot flushes related to my hormonal cycle.

Hot beds have led to very restless nights' sleep and whole weeks have been rendered dysfunctional by heat waves.

In short, the only remedy I have found (other than air-conditioning, swimming pools and shady creeks) is meditation on centring the mind beyond heat and the cooling breath (see cooling breath p.59) – try it, it works.

Fatigue

I have already given plenty of time to the description of fatigue in MS so I will just say that it's incapacitating and debilitating. Again, yoga and meditation have been the only things I have found that help this crippling symptom.

Going off line

Going off line is a term I coined early on in my journey with MS to describe losing function because it does often feel like that body part or function becomes disconnected from the mainframe.

It began with my legs when they would become more difficult to control and then extended through my body as more and more of my functions became difficult to control.

Sexual dysfunction

Another difficult topic but important and relevant to

the impact MS has on intimate relationships is sexual dysfunction. I have experienced both psychological and physical barriers to healthy sexual function.

Firstly, there is fatigue. It is hard to feel sexually motivated when you are constantly exhausted (ask any new mother).

Secondly there is the lack of self esteem and feeling attractive that goes hand in hand with being chronically disabled; as a friend said to me the other day, "I can't walk and piss my pants, how is that attractive?". I felt completely unattractive.

Then of course, there are the physical barriers like loss of sensitivity (loss of skin sensation affects the sexual organs as well and seems to be one of those symptoms that sticks), muscle spasms, muscle weakness and lack of flexibility due to spasticity – the options can be very limited, so forget the karma sutra!

Facial palsy

There are many people worse affected by this than me but it is noticeable, to me at least. I have become so used to the lopsidedness of my face that I almost didn't include it in these symptoms, until I was looking at photographs from my youth. I did have an even face. I don't now.

Groundhog days

As I have been writing this section of the book I have been re-experiencing the symptoms I have been writing about. I have even tasted the feelings of panic and crisis that comes with them.

It is almost like my mind–body complex has provided me with the symptoms so I can remember all the details and not miss a thing.

It has also served to remind me of how bizarre life is with MS and how normal life has become for me since yoga and meditation have come into my life – I feel such gratitude, compassion and more commitment than ever to share my story as honestly as possible.

Even the panic and crisis has served its purpose to remind me of the skills I have to deal with the emotional aspect of illness (and living generally); and in dealing with the emotional feelings of panic and crisis, the impact of the physical symptoms is minimised and sometimes eliminated.

We are all a breath away from difficulty but the skills I have learned over the last three years of yogic training really do work to help transform these difficulties into manageable life lessons to make us stronger.

The other gift of these Groundhog days is confirmation of my illness. I know that sounds strange but I have always experienced doubt about the reality of my illness.

"It's just in my head."

"I'm making it up."

"It's not nearly as bad as I'm making out."

These (and more) are all sentences that have gone through my mind on high rotation. Consequently, I haven't even been able to believe the evidence of my own body or that I deserved the help I was being given; constantly feeling guilty and undeserving.

The truth is, even one of the symptoms I have described here is unsettling; more than one, simultaneously, is annoying and a nuisance; all of them at once is completely debilitating and a complete pain in the backside (literally and metaphorically)!

One reason for this is the seeming impossible nature of the symptoms; another is the deceptive nature of the impact of the symptoms; and yet another is the attitude of doctors. I know neurologists see the very worst of neurological diseases but to tell someone their symptoms are relatively benign or insignificant compared to those of others with worse conditions, when the person is experiencing symptoms that question their underlying relationship with the world, is insensitive at best, and patronising and undermining at worst.

There are very few MS patients I have spoken with who haven't experienced this.

Meditation for headaches

- *Sit very still, as upright as you can (supported by cushions is good) or lying on your back if that is more comfortable.*
- *Slow your breath rate until you feel a stillness in your mind.*
- *Soften and broaden your vision, so that your mind relaxes.*
- *At the same time allow your face to relax.*
- *Gently close your eyes, keeping your gaze soft and your mind relaxed.*

- *As you sit in this stillness, you may feel it spread through your body.*
- *Encourage your body and your mind to let go*
- *with each breath out.*
- *Stay in this place for as long as you can and enjoy the feeling of space inside your mind.*
- *When you are ready to emerge, rub your hands together, cover your eyes.*
- *Open your eyes into the darkness of your palms, and then gently allow the light in while massaging your face and scalp.*

Take your time to return to the material world and take some of the stillness with you.

Core stability

- *The group of muscles that give the lower spine strength and stability, including the pelvic floor, transversus abdominus and the lumbar multifidus.*

*The **pelvic floor** is the sling of muscle at the base of the trunk — the muscle that keeps all your internal organs inside your abdominal cavity. To find it, breathe in and out deeply, and at the end of your out-breath, gently draw up the muscles from your pubic bone to the rear of your pelvis at the base of your trunk — that's the pelvic floor.*

A simple exercise to strengthen the pelvic floor:

- *contract the pelvic floor at the end of an out-*

breath,

- *Then breathe normally while you hold the contraction for six seconds.*
- *Repeat this six times, six times a day.*

The transversus abdominus and the lumbar multifidus *are the next keys to core stability strength. These are the deep internal muscles across your lower abdomen you'd suck in if you were trying to do up a tight pair of jeans They form a 'muscle corset' around the centre of your body. When these muscles are gently contracted you should be able to breathe, talk and laugh normally but your pelvis will be in a 'neutral' position.*

A simple exercise to begin recruiting the 'muscle corset':

- *make sure your back is straight and your feet are on the floor.*
- *take a deep breath in and at the end of the out-breath, gently contract the lower abdominal muscles*
- *Breathe normally, talk and laugh while you hold this contraction for ten seconds. Repeat ten times.*

Cooling breath
If you can roll your tongue

- *Roll your tongue and breathe in and out through the roll.*

- *Repeat until you feel coolness spread from the front to the back of the brain.*

If you cannot roll your tongue
- *Slightly open your mouth so there is a small gap between your teeth.*
- *Place your tongue behind the gap and breathe in and out through the gap in your teeth.*
- *Repeat until you feel coolness spread from the front to the back of the brain.*

The Road to Visualisation

SEPTEMBER 2004

The road to visualisation began in a hospital in Weston Supermare, UK.

The hospital had allocated funding for a 10 week Tai Chi trial for patients recovering from neurological injury. I had been attending weekly physiotherapy sessions at the hospital and my physiotherapist recommended me for the trial. I was already doing some yoga at home and the exercises the physiotherapist had recommended, but she also thought Tai Chi might be good for my balance.

I wish I could write to that physiotherapist now and thank her because those ten lessons in Tai Chi were the beginning of the recovery I am now enjoying. I remember very little actual Tai Chi from those lessons but three take-home messages are firmly engraved in my memory:

1. *do something every day, no matter how little, just do what you remember; you will either remember it because you loved it and therefore your body probably needs it or because you hate it and your body probably needs it; let the rest take care of itself.*
2. *you can move energy around your body with movement, think circles*
3. *If you can't do it, visualise!*

From my first physiotherapy session in hospital, when diagnosis was still a way off, I had begun doing a daily practice of physiotherapy exercises and yoga practices. Actually it was mostly just thinking about doing them because I couldn't do much physically. My core stability was likely to collapse at any given moment, so everything had to be done lying down or in my mind – I did, after all, have plenty of time to think!

After being discharged, I continued. Every day I did an odd combination of yoga and physiotherapy exercise, I did what I could remember and never felt sure I was doing the right thing, but I had to do something.

I had never been conscientious in my life: have never practiced, studied only enough to pass exams, written essays at the last minute and basically spent my entire life flying by the seat of my pants (pants through which had worn a seriously large hole). Yet here I was in the most debilitated state of my life, working harder than I ever had.

Even still I felt frustrated. I felt I wasn't doing enough; if only I could remember more; maybe I was doing the wrong things.

So when the Tai Chi instructor told me my body has its own intelligence and would remember what I need, it was like warm honey on a sore throat. Never before had my soul felt so soothed.

And the energy thing was a revelation I am still exploring. The idea we can move energy around the body, that we can visualise light and use the light in movement, was revolutionary to me but it felt so right. It was a seed planted still growing into a magnificent tree of knowledge and practice. My energy then, however, was somewhat blocked.

And visualisation? Wow! What a trip, to think you could visualise movement and the brain would respond as if the body had moved! The weird thing is, I had been thinking about physical movement I couldn't do since I was in hospital but just didn't think it was doing anything other than keeping me entertained.

However, he was very convincing and over the 10 weeks I watched stroke patients regaining movement in paralysed limbs due to visualisation. Sometimes the movement was marginal, the improvement subtle but when you can't move bits, anything is good. I couldn't quite get my head around it at the time but the idea stuck and the evidence in the patients around me was irrefutable.

So a few years later when I really couldn't move my bits and my teachers said 'don't worry, you can visualise', somewhere I knew I could.

A night at the pub

Meanwhile, at home I worked. My mobility improved so I started using my walking frame more than the wheelchair. Then, one night I had a fight with Matthew. I was furious and I was sick of being cooped up, being isolated, being dependent. I stormed out into the night; dark, raining, windy and cold.

The anger in my muscles propelled me up the road and into the nearest pub ... on my sticks! I hadn't walked so far since before hospital.

Pubs in Britain are friendly, people talk to strangers and people are interested. So, when a young Australian woman on Canadian crutches arrived out of the rain, people noticed.

I found a seat at the bar and bought my first half pint and before I knew it I was chatting. I was shouted drinks, even by the barman, and by closing time I was happily happy. The anger had been replaced by a strange sense of achievement; I had managed to do something by myself, again.

Now, I'm not suggesting that the answer to everyone's anger is to march off to the local pub on your crutches and have few pints of good English , but we all need to chat, to tell our story and hear other people's stories.

I didn't see any of those people again (other than the barman) and only returned to the pub once, a few months later just before returning to Australia. And my circumstances weren't changed by the sharing, but the act of sharing seemed to lighten my load and give me a different perspective.

And what amazed me was that a couple of months later, the barman remembered me and what I drank, so maybe hearing my story had also changed his perspective in some way (or he was a very good barman, or maybe both).

I revelled in stumbling home that night. I'm sure I looked completely drunk and I didn't mind at all because I was doing it myself.

There had been so many times over the previous few months when I looked drunk and wasn't, when people had judged a middle class woman dragging her legs and swaying to some unheard music, and I had cringed. Well, judge away!

It took a very long time to walk the short distance from the pub to my house and there was a lot of foot dragging and a lot of swaying but every step was bliss.

The next day I asked myself the question through a bleary mind: "If only I could marshal that anger to work for me without having to have a blue with my husband (a sentiment I'm sure he would have shared)."

The answer was determination. Anger became determination and from that day I worked harder and walked more; I knew I could do it.

By the time we left Britain in November, I was walking often without crutches and even taught a few days at my son's high school. They didn't know of 'probable MS' and no-one guessed there was anything wrong. The sense of achievement was exhilarating.

November/December

2004

We left Britain on the 19th November. There were so many mixed emotions as we packed up yet another house.

I felt sadness and grief for my children who were leaving social lives and acceptance they hadn't experienced in Australia. For me it was like leaving part of me in the UK; perhaps my innocence. I would never again live life without awareness of the impermanence of physical wellbeing. A chasm had settled between Matthew and I that we seemed unable to broach and he was leaving his family.

I was happy to be going 'home' but the uncertainty of our future back in Australia and the unresolved pain of the life we were leaving behind made the happiness fragile and brittle. How would I be able to face my family and friends as a disabled person?

Wanting to take advantage of being overseas, we decided to spend a couple of weeks in Thailand on the way back to Australia. I couldn't really camp and we couldn't really travel a lot so for the first in our family's life, we stayed in a resort – it was fabulous!

During that holiday I did things I never thought I would do again; snorkelled, was in and out of boats and swam.

There were down days and moments when I needed to be helped in and out of cars. The local restaurant would order a taxi (their cousin) to drive us back to the hotel when we asked for the bill after the first night when I couldn't walk.

But there was hope and I was living. I smiled at the world and the world smiled back. At the airports I needed a wheelchair but that was no big deal, I just smiled and laughed and allowed myself to be wheeled, and I was wheeled and the people smiled back.

We visited several temples, one with the Buddha's teeth, and all with a sense of calm and generosity we in the west don't seem to be able to manifest. My favourite was the Tiger Temple, a vispassna retreat built around a huge tiger paw print in the upper part of a cave.

We bought a brass Buddha, were given handmade bracelets and I bought my first mala (a handmade string of beads used to chant mantras – one repetition of mantra per bead). Now I could really begin chanting compassion.

I went into the cave and found myself surrounded by statues of sitting monks, and then out of the corner of my eye I spied a particularly life like statue. I looked again and the 'statue' broke into a huge smile and we both laughed. He invited me to visit the paw print and then to sit with him. It felt so special.

I began chanting on my mala, a beautiful practice I continue to this day.

Again I found my perspective change. Thai people smile, they seem to smile all the time. Maybe not everyone all the time but most, most of the time, and it changed the way I experienced life – it really is completely different with a smile and a laugh. *Try it: just smile, for no reason other than you're alive, and see what happens.*

The three-year old who wanted to be a yogi

Once upon a time a three year old girl sat mesmerised in front of a television screen. What was on the screen? Was it Play School or Sesame Street or another of the myriad of children's television? No, it was the daily yoga routine of Swami Saraswati, an exotic Indian yogi living in Australia.

The little girl thought the yogi was the most beautiful woman she had ever seen and wanted to be a yogi just like her. She practised positions like the lotus, shoulder stand and sitting twists and putting her foot behind her head; and felt a strange sense of peace.

Time went on and the little girl went to school, and stopped practicing but she never stopped sitting cross legged and always loved going upside down.

As an adult the girl was constantly drawn to yoga classes, sporadically doing her own practice at home. It felt so familiar and natural but she never found that something she was looking for. Of course, she didn't know she was looking for a feeling she had had when she was three, in fact she had forgotten she even had a feeling when she was three. She just knew that yoga felt right but not right enough.

Then one day she went to a new yoga class and found the feeling again…

Coming Home

2005

I arrived back in Australia in the heat of summer. By the time we got through customs I could hardly sit up, let alone walk. My brother met us at Sydney airport and I could feel his eyes watching everything I did.

I had left Sydney a seemingly healthy young woman and returned twelve months later hardly able to walk, and although my family received regular updates from Britain, I don't think you can ever accurately describe that level of disability. There was more controlled shock when I arrived at my sister's.

Within a week I had recovered some of the wellbeing I had experienced before leaving Britain and we returned to Braidwood, into the house we had rented from the UK. Matthew had moved our belongings and now it was time to unpack – ugh!

Heat and grief combined to limit my ability to function – the fatigue was indescribable. I noticed everything I couldn't do. I continued stretching and yoga-ing every day. It had become a part of my day by then. We unpacked as much as we could and began preparing Gabriel for boarding school.

He was still determined to try boarding school and so, with heavy hearts, we labelled and shopped and labelled some more. A few weeks after moving into our new house I was again saying goodbye, this time to my son. God, it was horrible – gut-wrenching grief.

For two terms we drove the hour to Goulburn every Friday to pick him up from the station and every Sunday we returned him to the station to go back to school. This alone was exhausting and, thankfully, we all decided it wasn't worth the pain.

Meanwhile, Grace settled into the local school, and Nicola, who was then 19 months-old, began to walk. Matthew commuted over an hour every day between our home in Braidwood and his new job in Canberra, and a semblance of normality descended.

When the fatigue hit I would lie on the couch and read to Nicola. When the symptoms hit I would lie on the couch and read to Nicola. When I couldn't read we would have a nap.

On a school excursion to the District Swimming Carnival I happened to mention I was a maths tutor and suddenly I was tutoring again. I loved it.

At the same time, I started to speak to publishers about writing textbook material again. After a few months and several samples, I finally had an agreement with a publisher to write teachers' websites for a series of science textbooks (four books, and every chapter needed multiple choice, short answers, fill in the blanks and extension questions, as well as tests).

I also began a regime of acupuncture, Chinese herbs and restricted diet (see *Diet box* p.77). The acupuncture seemed to subtly reprogram my entire body and the diet, while depressingly difficult to maintain, felt clean and virtuous. Strangely, I got self-esteem from depriving myself of all my favourite food! The mind is a bizarre thing.

Then halfway through the year my acupuncturist recommended the Dru yoga class she attended, saying I would love it. (see *What is Dru?* Appendix)

She drove me to my first class and she was right, I loved it from the very first moment. I still remember the feeling of deep comfort mid-twist during Energy Block Release 7 (one of the key Dru movement sequences), 'like slipping into a warm bath'. It combined everything I had been doing instinctively for myself, with some extra bits thrown in.

I loved the classes so much; it seemed natural to begin doing some Dru through the day.

I began becoming more aware of my posture, remembering the steps going into Tadasana while standing in the kitchen or in a bank queue, and practicing do-in in the shower in the morning (see *do-in* and *Tadasana* p.79). Even these small practices carried some of the energy of the Dru class I loved.

As I became more familiar with other practices I began to practice them at home, too. The neck movements from Energy Block Release Sequence 1 (see *Neck*

movements p.80) became a regular, as did some of the beautiful lying down spinal twists from Energy Block Release 7 (still one of my favourites to savour p.82).

At the same time I was becoming more aware of my breath. Teaching breath as an integral part of movement is essential in Dru Yoga. We are taught to synchronise movement with the breath, giving the movement power and grace while attuning it to one's own natural rhythm.

It seemed quite natural for me so I started to experiment doing it with every day ordinary movements at home, and the difference it makes to breathe in synchronicity with your body is astonishing. (See **Breathing with movement** p.80)

Yoga and acupuncture really started to make me more aware of my body. The diet regime and the herbs and the needles were having a calming effect on my poor digestive system, and both the yoga and the needles were improving my general energy levels. I walked with my sticks less often, my balance improved and I had more stamina.

As the year progressed I noticed I felt more and more of the feeling I loved so much in the Dru class when I did these little bits of practice. It is difficult to describe that feeling and I am unwilling to try, except to say it was like coming home. Imagine feeling like you were coming home just from doing some do-in and a few neck twists – awesome.

I had been tutoring maths and science all year, and had begun writing the website, while parenting my three children. The two older kids said I did more in a day than most people without MS, although I did spend a lot of time resting when they were at school and Nicola was read to a lot – it was the only thing I could do to entertain her when the MS fatigue arrived.

Diet box

Do's
- *Lots of vegetables, lots of different colours*
- *Zinc e.g. oysters*
- *Deep sea fish (fish oil)*
- *Rice*
- *Almonds*
- *Fresh juices*
- *Berries*

Don'ts
- *Saturated fats*
- *Dairy*
- *Meat*
- *Eggs*
- *Reduced caffeine (I stopped drinking coffee every day, and eventually stopped altogether and drank mostly non-caffeinated tea)*
- *Raw food (I ate some fruit but salads really disrupted my digestion)*
- *Processed food*
- *Wheat*

I still keep to this diet as much as I can, although I eat eggs and supplement with Vitamin D.

Do-in

Do in is a light rhythmical tapping of the body, using your finger tips to stimulate the body's energy system.

It can be done all over the body and when I first started a regular Dru practice I gave myself a full body do-in every day.

It was like waking up my body and giving myself a full body treatment in just a few minutes; one of the many practices I have learnt in Dru I call self-nurturing practices. These are practices we can do for ourselves that give us the nurturing we would otherwise pay people money to do for us.

On the other hand, you can give Do-in to specific parts of the body for specific effects.

Chest Do-in and sternum circling

An effective and simple daily practice is to tap with the fingertips all over the chest. This stimulates the thymus gland, which in turn stimulates the immune system — a great practice for winter and warding off colds etc.

Combine this with sternum circling for a quick stimulation and relaxing of the whole chest area, including the diaphragm.

(Your sternum is your breast bone and begins

at the bottom where your ribs meet. The diaphragm is the flat muscle at the base of the sternum and one of the main muscles in-breathing.)

Begin circling the base of your sternum with your middle finger. I f you come across any tender bits notice them and move on, no judgement. Continue on in this way up the sternum until you reach the collarbone then repeat a few times.

This practice releases tension you might be holding in the diaphragm and hence expands your breath, stimulating points along the sternum, further supporting the cardio-pulmonary reflex arc.

Tadasana

Tadasana is the first Sanskrit word I learnt and still stands in my lexicon as one of the most important concepts in yoga.

Tadasana roughly translates to Mountain and is the art of standing with energy, strength and purpose of a mountain. It brings stillness and dignity into something we all do many, many times in a day.

And whenever I remember to stand like a mountain in my daily life, something ripples through my awareness and I feel different.

The essence is to have your feet under your hips, your spine in alignment, shoulders relaxed, head sitting on top your spine and your whole body relaxed into this posture; your mind completely present in the moment.

I imagine a golden cord coming out of my spine and holding me so my feet rest on the ground and my skeleton falls naturally in alignment.

Breathing with movement

There are three basic principles to breathing with movement:

- *Breathe in when you are unfolding the body or lifting and breathe out when you are folding the body over*
- *When twisting, breath in and lengthen, breathe out when you twist and breathe in to come back to centre*
- *Breathe out when you are actively stretching a muscle and breathe in to rest, (particularly useful with hamstrings)*

Neck movements

Neck Roll

- *Sit or stand with a straight back and relaxed shoulders.*
- *Focus your attention on your chin, breathe in and lengthen your neck, upwards.*
- *On the breath out lower the chin towards your chest; allow the movement to begin at the base of the neck.*
- *Breathe in and raise the chin until you can*

look up very slightly; again, the movements begins at the base of the neck.

- *Create a wave-like motion of the neck vertebrae as you repeat the movement two more times.*

Head Tilt

- *Breathe in and lengthen your neck upwards.*
- *On your out-breath, tilt your head to the right so your right ear moves out to the side (imagine the vertebrae shearing to the right) and down towards the right shoulder.*
- *Breathe in and imagine a string pulling your left ear up as you raise your head; imagine the vertebrae stacking from the base of the neck.*
- *Repeat to the left side.*
- *Imagine the space between the vertebrae expanding and the muscles around the base of the neck lengthening as you repeat this to each side, twice more.*

Neck Rotation

- *On your breath in, lengthen your neck, upwards.*
- *Breathe out and turn your head to the right as far as is comfortable, keeping your chin parallel with the floor.*
- *Breathe in as your head returns to the front and repeat to the left side.*
- *Imagine the vertebrae rotating one by one*

and the muscles around the neck letting go of any tension as you repeat this movement two more times to each side.

EBR7 spinal twists

There are two fabulous things about these spinal twists: one, you can do them lying down; and two, they leave your spine feeling spacious and your chest open.

- *Lay on your right side with your legs at right angles.*
- *Relax your body as you breathe out.*
- *Stretch your arms out in front of you with the palms facing.*
- *As you breathe in, raise your left arm over your body towards the ground on the left side, opening your chest and following your arm with your soft gaze.*
- *Only take your arm as far as is comfortable, ensuring your right shoulder stays on the ground.*
- *Breathing out as your bring your arm back over so the left palm rests on the upturned right palm.*
- *Repeat two more times on the right then roll over and repeat on the left side.*

The other twist is called the spiral.
- *Lay on your right side with your legs at right angles.*
- *As you breathe in take your left arm over*

your head so you trace a circle around your body.

- *Allow your spine to stretch out.*
- *Imagine your spine becoming more spacious.*
- *Breathe out over the second half of the circle.*
- *Repeat this circular motion two more times, then repeat on the left side.*

My Father's Passing

SEPTEMBER 2005

One afternoon in early September 2005, not long after we had moved into a new house, we got a call that was to shatter the fragile equilibrium I had established – my father had suffered a major heart attack. The advice from my family was to wait before driving up to Sydney but within days he had suffered further attacks, causing irreparable damage to his heart muscle.

We loaded the family in to the car and drove to Sydney. I had just come out of an acupuncture appointment and was determined to retain some of the peace I had gained so I sat in the back and breathed all the way down (or up depending on your geographic sensibilities) the highway to North Shore Hospital. It really did make a difference to my state of mind.

When we arrived at North Shore Hospital my father said a small sentence that still resonates to this day. He had been slipping in out of a delirious state but when he was present he was really, really present, and as Nicola was on his tummy giving the kind of cuddle only Nicola can give (Nicola loves everyone and assumes everyone loves her and cuddles with that supreme confidence and abandon), he said "You've got a lovely little family Lyn".

Regardless of the criticism that had happened before and the stuff that came up after, I can always remember that small sentence reminding me he did notice.

Buoyed by my success at controlling the emotional panic that was threatening to overwhelm me, I continued breathing through the next week of daily hospital visits. The tension amongst my siblings and mother was excruciating as we waited but breathing made it seem possible.

My father turned a corner with the help of cutting edge drugs and was moved to a ward in a hospital near his home. That was my last task before returning to Braidwood; overseeing the transfer. When the transfer was complete and another family member was on their way to replace me, it was time to go home.

We both knew this might be the last time we saw each other, something I could feel and see it in his eyes. As I said goodbye I knew it might really be goodbye but I couldn't say, 'I love you'. As I walked away I hoped beyond hope that I had said everything I needed to say. I hoped I had said it before: I hoped he knew.

Sure enough, a short time later he returned home from hospital and within a few days, my father passed away in his own chair, at home.

Another trip to Sydney for the funeral followed. The funeral was a celebration of his life and we were all gracious through its organising and the day itself, particularly my mother, who was just beautiful. Three siblings spoke about different aspects of his life; my eldest brother about the early years and the history; by middle brother about the other love of his life, the boat; and me about how him and how he affected people. It was perfect.

It is hard to explain what happens to a family when a parent dies. It is like a lid is removed from a pressure cooker and all the bubbles of discontent from childhood are free to rise to the surface and overflow. During the funeral and immediately after we were the epitome of cooperation, but over the next six months we unravelled and, well, we all went a little mad.

Although I felt a sense of loss when he passed, the emotional numbness of the previous few years prevented me from really expressing the grief. I was still in shock and this added to it. The main emotion was a sense of relief that he was no longer suffering.

A friend of mine recently spoke to me about her own grief. People had told her how hard grief was but she hadn't found it that difficult and I had experienced the same feeling. However, like my friend, it was easy because I hadn't actually allowed myself to feel the grief and it expressed itself through my madness.

My father was the patriarch in my family and his passing left a huge gulf. He had been a strong disciplinarian and conservative in his values, so when he passed I felt this huge weight of judgement lift from my shoulders. I wanted to rebel and feel free to do anything. Yet I felt hamstrung by the responsibilities of parenthood and marriage and chronic illness.

I think if I felt angry at any time during my journey with MS this was it. I still couldn't just be me. Even writing about it now, I can sense the angst I felt at the time, the inner rage against the machine. But I didn't rage and be honest; I turned it in on myself. And so even though I experienced a brief period of wellness practicing Dru every day (*The first spark of splendour* opposite), it didn't last because the core was rotten.

The first spark of splendour, January 2006

I had continued attending yoga classes through the second half of 2005 and came to love it more and more, so just before Christmas I borrowed my yoga teacher's copy of the recently released Dru DVD and became addicted.

First there's Mansukh, who I am sure could inspire the most slothful of us to change our diet, and begin doing yoga and meditation.

Then there's the rest of the DVD, with short manageable activations and yoga sequences for beginners and more advanced students. Morning, afternoon, bedtime, partners, kiddies, meditation and nutrition – like a one-stop shop for budding yogis. Nothing too earnest or too beautiful or too sweaty, just the understated elegance of stillness in motion (and no, they're not paying me to say this).

Anyway, I started getting up at five in the morning to practice; sometimes practicing for an hour and a half before Nicola (then 2½) awoke. My energy was amazing. I remember feeling the space between the cells expanding after some sessions, like the atoms were somehow spinning faster. My mind felt so clear and creative.

It was a taste, and while it didn't last because, as I said before, the core was rotten, the feeling of those couple of months stayed in my memory as an example of how I could feel.

The Slippery Slope

2006

After the initial burst of energy in the first couple of months of 2006, the slide began. I started to feel different symptoms and acupuncture was starting to be less effective. And I started to feel really tired again. During one needle session, I felt so tired I could have easily just fallen asleep on the table and not woken.

I wasn't suicidal and I wasn't depressed and I didn't want to leave my family; I just felt *so* tired. These days when I get tired in this way I rest in meditation but then I didn't have such wisdom and just wanted to go to sleep for a very long time.

Then came the flu. It was just a flu to everyone else but I couldn't cough (absent coughing reflex is an MS symptom) and the phlegm sat in my lungs and did what phlegm does – grow bugs.

What followed was a weekend of thrashing fever and agonising pain, and of course no doctors. Off to my GP on Monday, feeling like I had been run over by a bus but a little better – at least the bus had moved on.

The doctor gave me a prescription and took a blood sample, "just in case". The following morning I received a phone call from same GP while I was hanging washing on the line.

"How are you?" he asked.

"Fine, just hanging washing on the line. Why?" I asked.

"I have just had a phone call from the pathologist," he said, "suggesting you should be in hospital on intravenous antibiotics."

I was so used to feeling like excrement, I didn't take it seriously. It is also difficult to tell the difference between MS and what normal illness is, and periodically I do get thoroughly sick of going to doctors.

I had turned my own corner and didn't need hospital but it took weeks to recover, even with the antibiotics. The flu exaggerated the slide that had already begun. I remember feeling angry and guilty and thinking, "but I was doing everything right, it's not fair". I felt like the deterioration was my fault but I couldn't do any more.

I was too tired to resume my daily appointment with the digital Mansukh and, while I was still getting to class, my practice was sliding.

My yoga teacher gave me a copy of the Dru Bhagavad Gita and I started to read it. I remember thinking how I couldn't possibly be like this wise person but I really, really wanted to be.

Over time, I also stopped acupuncture and herbs.

I had started seeing a Chinese doctor in Canberra but it was such a long way and it was so expensive to maintain the weekly appointments, and a friend had to drive me and look after Nicola. It was just so difficult.

And conveniently, at this time, Nicola decided it was time to give up her afternoon sleep. At first I struggled and felt exhausted just by the effort of trying to get her to sleep. Then I remembered a practice I had learnt at an earlier Dru class – 'legs up the wall'. "Twenty minutes was equal to two hours sleep" the presenter said. She was right, Nicola loved doing it with me so at least some element of sanity returned, even if it looked a little weird. (***Legs up the wall*** p.97).

At the same time the fallout from my father's death the year before was hitting my siblings and myself, and I think we were all a little mad.

Yet even in the middle of this turmoil there were brief moments of positivity and sanity that were to give me foundations for the next phase of my life.

Somehow I had been referred to an occupational therapist who then referred me on to a government agency supporting disabled people back into the workforce. A support officer visited my house to see what they could do.

I felt very undeserving and quite guilty for accepting this help because I didn't think I was that disabled. These feelings of guilt and unworthiness sat and festered with other similar feelings but were mitigated to some extent by a deep sense of gratitude at the generosity still left in the world.

On seeing my work arrangement (my desk was a coffee table while I sat on the floor) and hearing of my symptoms she was mildly horrified that I should be working in such conditions and began thinking how her agency could help. The priority for her was a desk and the idea of voice activated software to help me write when my hands became dysfunctional.

I was shocked that someone would want to help me in this way and didn't quite believe it was actually going to happen or that I deserved it, but it did. Funding was approved, and appointments were made to see the ergonomic office-ware specialists and a software consultant.

Within a couple of months I had a desk that could be wound up and down to accommodate a wheelchair (I hated it at the time but it was inspired forethought), an ergonomic stand for my laptop, foot rest and a desk chair. Then came my Dragon (voice activated software) and Dragon training. I loved my Dragon and while I didn't need to use it all the time, later it was my life saver.

In hindsight I am so grateful to those people for understanding the degenerative nature of MS. At the time I could only see the present (well, I wasn't actually even in the present) and was too scared to think about what might happen in the future but their support enabled me to continue functioning when I wouldn't have been able to otherwise.

Their intervention in my life also helped me to discover a very important lesson about the descent into disability – *accept the aides!* Life with a disability may not be what I had wanted in my life and accepting the use of aides does require an acknowledgement of one's disability but as I learnt time and again, using the aides ensures far greater independence and quality of life than battling and struggling without them. And ultimately, the psychological gift is acceptance.

Sanity came in the form of a Dru seminar on yoga and meditation for managing emotional crisis. Yep, that's me. My yoga teacher in Braidwood and some fellow students were driving into Canberra so I joined them.

One of the presenters lead a beautiful meditation called the Blue Mist Meditation, still one of my favourites, and I spoke with him afterwards. His name was Andrew and he recommended I come to a meditation retreat at the end of the year, suggested we do some telephone mentoring and mentioned I seemed to instinctively know what was good for me. I didn't know at the time but he was to become one of the most important figures in my recovery.

We weren't able to do the mentoring, I wasn't able to go the meditation retreat, and the day wasn't enough to halt the slide in my practice and my wellbeing, but it was another taste of something I felt instantly connected with.

I had developed a spasmodic ringing in my ears that would just come and ring for a bit and then leave, always when I was the most tired. It still does.

And I was getting new visual disturbances where my vision just wouldn't clear. You know when you've had too many drinks and your vision goes blurry and you try really hard to make it clear but it won't happen (sorry to the non-drinkers, you will just have to imagine and be thankful you have never experienced it)? That's what it was like, without the alcohol, and sometimes first thing in the morning.

Once again, I had that same spinning out of control feeling, as though everything around me was about to crash. Looking back I can recognise the symptoms of an MS exacerbation and that is one of them.

Every day seemed to be an exercise in holding on, getting through the symptoms and feeling so tired. I would find excuses for symptoms to have appeared; I was hot or tired or getting the flu again or, or, or … anything to fool my mind out of the thought I might be going there again, yet wanting to complete everything just in case I was; working even harder to imaginary, self-created deadlines.

I was in the mode expectant mothers sometimes enter just before the baby is born, trying to get all the nesting done before the baby comes. For me it was like getting everything done before the disaster strikes. I still do that.

I was tutoring, writing and parenting, all while trying to pretend I wasn't getting worse. I was trying to be 'Super Cripple'.

Then in July 2006 I was driving home at night and my vision went. It could have been a mistake – it was night and I could have just had a lapse in concentration. When getting changed at home the same thing happened and this time I fell over. I recognised a feeling of familiarity – this had happened before but for some reason I had chosen not to notice. The mind is such a powerful entity.

Time to see my doctor.

Legs up the wall (modified version)

This practice originates from the restorative series of inverted postures and I have even modified it further. I was unable to rest with my legs literally up the wall due to my ever decreasing muscle strength, fatigue and tight lower back and hamstrings, so I put my legs over a chair and it still works and Nicola loved doing it.

At the same time every day we would line our chairs up together, her child-sized chair and my 'growed-up' one, get into position and then rest for as long as she could – usually about twenty minutes. This is what we did.

- *Lie down on your side with your bottom at the base of the chair and your legs at right angles.*
- *Roll over on to your back and rest the lower half of your leg over the seat of the chair.*
- *Cover yourself with a blanket, close your eyes and rest.*
- *That's it!*

- *When you are ready to come out of the posture roll back on to your side and rest a few moments there before getting up — small children will start chatting immediately but they will be sufficiently relaxed to wait for mum or dad to chill.*

It really does feel like two hours rest.

The Relapse

JULY 2006

My condition had deteriorated while I was still pretending everything was fine. I went to the doctor and with one glance he was already talking about steroids – a common treatment for relapsing MS patients, designed to reduce the inflammation in the brain – even before I told him about my symptoms.

What was funny was that I had convinced myself I was fine, but as soon as he recognised I wasn't, so did I. The exhaustion I had felt, both from MS fatigue and trying so hard to stay upright flooded my mind and again I just wanted to go to sleep for a very long time.

I thought I had walked into the surgery, which was next door to my house, but later when questioned by my husband the doctor said I was barely walking, more from determination than anything else. I was shocked at the time, but when I look back now with the detachment of time, I realise he was right. I had dragged myself to the doctor on my sticks, as I had been dragging myself around for days possibly weeks, determined to 'walk'.

My doctor ordered the steroids on the Friday and rang over the weekend to make the appointment for me to come in to the local hospital on Monday and begin the treatment. This caused deeper shock on two fronts: first there was no time to procrastinate and second if he is ringing me on the weekend it must be bad.

The procedure takes about an hour and a half, and involves having a canula inserted, connected to the bag and the steroids are dripped into the blood stream. The patient goes home and comes back the next day for three more days – or at least that's the plan.

Unfortunately things didn't go to plan and I reacted to the steroids. Rather than going home, I was admitted and I don't really know what happened next. The steroids dose was halved so my reaction the next day was only minor but my MS symptoms deteriorated.

When I was discharged on the Friday, I couldn't walk. I couldn't sit up, I couldn't shower, take myself to the toilet, and sometimes I could barely use my arms and hands to eat, or swallow or talk clearly. Sometimes I was so tired, I couldn't even hold my head up.

As I sit here writing now, it occurs to me that perhaps I just gave up fighting; perhaps I was just too tired. The shock deepened.

The best thing was I had stopped smoking and haven't had a cigarette since!

Then came the helpers. Once again our home was

barraged by people we didn't know, asking very personal questions that were difficult to answer, but really, really wanting to help.

I can't explain what it is like to have your home suddenly become an open thoroughfare, even when it is for people to shower you or look after you and your family. It is like suddenly you have no boundaries, no privacy. The business of you and your family are open for the world to see. In any circumstance this is difficult but in a small town where you sneeze and the town says, "Bless you", it is very confronting.

Under the guidance of two angels of mercy, a care plan was established, disability allowance was applied for and long term applications were made for equipment and care.

I came home from hospital in a manual wheelchair but it had to be returned and so another was found, although I couldn't wheel it very far because my arms were so weak. I was completely dependent on others for everything; I couldn't even go outside without somebody wheeling me.

Weeks went by where the only people I spoke to were those who were paid to visit the house for some MS reason or another. Of course, I spoke to the children and I had rudimentary conversations with Matthew but there was no intimacy in my life.

I think for a while I stopped trying. I felt so lost. I tried to go to Dru class but it was sporadic and then the classes stopped. I had started seeing a counsellor and she was lovely but I felt like I had lost the Dru personal practice that had come to be my best friend and I felt bereft.

I felt like I had lost contact with the one thing in my life (outside of my children) that really felt like me.

I finally felt like I had lost everything and fell into a clinical depression. My world felt so bleak.

I was still tutoring, still mothering to some degree but I felt nothing … nothing except fear and loneliness.

The emotions of MS

This may be the hardest chapter of my journey to write but I need to write it to put the next part of my journey into context.

Multiple Sclerosis is called the mystery disease, not just because the case is unknown but also because the day to day presentation of the illness is highly unpredictable, for both patients and doctors. There are general trends and patterns in fatigue and heat sensitivity that enable both doctors and people with MS to establish care plans, but get a room full of people with MS and you will have as many different sets of symptoms as there are people in the room.

In addition to the diversity of symptoms and clinical presentation there is the diversity in doctors opinions of what is and isn't caused by MS. There have been several symptoms and patterns that doctors have told me were nothing to do with MS, yet when I have spoken with other MS patients I have discovered they are actually common symptoms or patterns.

One that immediately comes to mind is the exaggeration of my symptoms, particularly fatigue, in the week preceding my period and the couple of days around ovulation. At least one doctor has told me that it is nothing to do with MS, but during an open chat session with a group of MS patients, several of the women expressed the same pattern, and since then more women with MS have said the same thing.

There have also been published surveys discussing the cyclic nature of some women's MS symptoms and a possible explanation – the exacerbation may occur as a consequence of increased body temperature during ovulation and premensis, with some women affected more than others.

Add this to months, sometimes years, of seemingly idiosyncratic symptoms appearing sporadically, sometimes resulting in misdiagnosis, and often with both patient and doctor thinking of hypochondriacs with prescription anti depressants (this seems to occur less these days, with more awareness and MRI technology but it still happens). It is little wonder MS patients feel confused, disempowered and can tend towards cynicism, even tipping into bitterness, regarding our condition.

We lose faith in our body because we can no longer trust it will do what we want it to do and (progressive patients excluded) we don't know from day to day, sometimes even hour to hour, how our body will respond. The illusion we used to have of knowing what tomorrow will bring is lost.

Depression is often both a symptom and a side effect of MS. This is all on top of any pre-existing psychology.

And for many, seething anger.

The props our society uses to give identity, whether we judge them as superficial or not, are material successes: physical beauty; indicators of youth; health and mobility; independence; career success; wealth or at least security; winning; and a mortgage, 2.2 children and two cars in the garage.

MS knocks out some, if not all of these props, for most of us, indefinitely, with little hope of recovery under the spectre of deterioration.

In addition, there is stigma attached to disability and disease, as if we have done something wrong to cause our illness. People feel uncomfortable and tend to keep their distance. For many people I was not only crippled but deaf and stupid as well.

During the months immediately after the exacerbation, I could only see a life of disability and loss. I could only see my life deteriorating. There was little intimacy in my life, and there were few people I had conversations with who were not paid to be with me or paying me to tutor them.

Doctors have said to me that MS is not too bad as far as neurological diseases go. At least it's not terminal. Well, I can tell you, I was 41 with three children between 3 and 13 when I was in the wheelchair, being bathed every day by strangers. I didn't think I would ever get out of the wheelchair, I looked at my future and saw forty years of increasing cognitive dysfunction, incontinence, isolation, increasing dependence, pain etc, etc, etc, etc and it didn't feel 'not too bad' to me.

Every time someone said to me, "at least it's not terminal", I silently wished it was. There were moments during that time when I envied people with terminal illnesses; at least they had an end to their suffering.

Depression.

Numbness.

I remember hearing my daughter cry and not feeling any emotional response.

I felt isolated and lost.

The Turn Around

LATE 2006

Two things happened that turned my life around.

The first thing was being served notice on the house we were living in. I know that sounds strange but sometimes a good kick up the backside is exactly what we need to move us out of the negative space we are in, and this was exactly what the notice to move was for me.

We were able to get the house next door, which I had been coveting since the day we moved in to the house we were in. It was a beautiful old double-brick house, built in the times of high ceilings and bay windows.

Despite moving next door, it was the most chaotic move I have experienced, and I have moved a few times! We were funded to have removalists but they did a lot less than we thought so we were stuck with doing a lot more packing than we were expecting on the day of the move. I was able to get out of the wheelchair and use my sticks for very short distances by then, so I was able to do enough to be a nuisance, constantly being told to sit down and get out of the way.

Finally, Matthew asked someone to wheel me over to the new house and make sure I didn't do anything. I was getting so tired I could hardly keep my head up but I was determined to be useful. I wonder what I was trying to prove.

While we never got unpacked properly and never properly settled, we lived there happily for just over two years. The house seemed to open up to us and start to breathe as soon as we moved in, despite our chaos.

The local Catholic Church offered to pay for the old house to be cleaned and I was overwhelmed by their generosity. It took an incredible load off our minds to know we didn't have to think about cleaning the house. Then I rang the carpet cleaners and discovered the church had already booked them. Once again, I cried with gratitude. An auspicious beginning

The second thing that happened was I rang the Dru office. I don't know why I rang, perhaps it was about the phone mentoring with Andrew or perhaps it was the meditation retreat but whatever it was I am grateful. The generosity and warmth in the voice at the other end of the phone was a lifeline for me.

I wasn't feeling that much warmth from people I knew at the time but from someone I didn't know it was unparalleled. We talked for a while and she suggested visualising. I was too tired to visualise but my contact with my practice was regained and I started to read the Gita again. I felt there was something in there for me if only I could find it.

I also started to dip into the *Little Book of Happiness* again. It's amazing how much good stuff is in such a little book.

These may seem small things for someone who had been doing an hour practice a day but to me they were significant reconnections to a way of thinking and being that had made MS seem manageable; where the emphasis wasn't on the things I had lost but on the value of compassion and detachment, and the peace that subsequently arises.

Around that time a friend offered to drive me into Canberra to the Chinese doctor and mind Nicola. It was such a generous gift and made such a difference to my life, particularly my digestion.

I can't tell you how bad the herbs smelled when I boiled them each day. The smell went through the whole house. My family was disgusted and warned their friends or apologised if they happened to come in when the herbs were cooking. Gabriel and Grace couldn't even go near the pot to smell them, and their odour was only exceeded by their taste, but I took them religiously, two times a day.

My mind even started to look forward to them. Weird what the mind gets used to if it's therapeutic.

Slowly my digestion started to improve, and my mobility started to improve a little also. I went to see another neurologist in Canberra. He suggested I think about taking anti-depressants.

I conferred with my counsellor and my GP. I told them about my emotional numbness and they both said, while they were reticent to recommend anti-depressants, in my case they thought it was a good plan.

Another barrier to cross for me; I had always been so judgemental of anti-depressants as an answer to depression. I had thought real solutions needed to be found to the fundamental cause of the depression rather than the band-aid of anti-depressants. Yet here I was being recommended to take them by people whose view I respected. How could I get my head around that?

Then a friend talked to me about her experience with anti-depressants. Her life had seemed out of control and overwhelming, and it was getting darker and heavier. She took anti-depressants for a year and they lifted the cloud, enabling her to regain a sense of control and navigate the life issues causing her to feel out of control.

They weren't the answer to her problems; they just lightened the load so she could find the answer, herself. At the end of the year she stopped taking them and hasn't needed to since.

Here was someone I respected, who had used anti-depressants in a responsible way and they had worked. It seemed this was another 'belief' I needed to let go: a cage I had carefully constructed, "anti-depressants are bad" that was preventing me from being present in my own situation as it was.

It appears to me that much of my journey with MS has been about letting go of the conditions and preconceptions I had put on the world. I was learning to assess each situation, each day, for its own merit rather than from the perspective of the 'rules' I had set up in my mind.

When the anti-depressants lifted the dark cloud of depression, I started to see the beauty in the world again and I started to live with what I had rather than what I had lost. The natural optimism I have felt through my life started to surface, and the love deeper than life I felt for my children meant I could see something worth living for again.

Ultimately, I discovered the only way to live with MS was to accept my condition, whatever it might be on any given day, and find a deeper sense of identity; a deeper reason to love; a purpose and identity independent of my material wellbeing.

My son, the joker

Being dependent on a wheelchair for mobility restricts movement outside the home to people willing and able to push the chair, and in Braidwood that meant strength to get chair up and down steep curbs or over cracks in the pavement. This meant relying on my son or my husband, which meant hardly ever.

Gabriel (and sometimes Matthew) never quite got his head around the vulnerability of someone in a wheelchair – how it might feel when the chair is pulled back going up hill.

One day Gabriel was pushing me down the main street and my daughters walking beside me. We were all talking and laughing and then my son also began walking beside me. We were going quite fast and laughing and then I realised I was looking at my son; if I was looking at him, who had control of my chair? No one. "I was wondering how long it would take you to realise. You should see the look on your face. Hahaha...."

Needless to say, he didn't do it again.

The Power
Chair – Freedom,
Yaaaaaaaayyyyyyyyy!
NOVEMBER 2006

The most fabulous thing in the world happened with the serendipity that appears to have characterised my journey.

A woman whose daughter had passed away donated her power chair to Queanbeyan Hospital and one of the amazing women who were looking after me offered it to me. Another of the amazing women looking after me facilitated the handover and Matthew picked it up from the hospital in time for me to go to the Majors Creek Folk Festival.

Freedom!!!!!!!!!!!!!!!!

I can buy my own tampons!

I hadn't realised until the festival how disempowered I had felt by my lack of mobility and independence. Here I was being able to go to the toilet, get a drink (my chair had a cup holder), go shopping through the festival market…all by myself. I felt like all my Christmases had come at once, the cat that licked the cream, on top of the world and all the other euphemisms for damn fine, all in one go. Yeehah!

Oh, and another bonus, Nicola loved to sit on it.

From the day I received the chair, I went out nearly every day, as long as it wasn't raining. I felt so free and was frequently seen hurtling down the street in full laughter with Nicola laughing equally on my lap. It's the little things in life, and buying your own tampons is one of them.

The next hurdle was the lack of access to just about every business in town. There was one cafe and one supermarket where entry and navigation was easy. The rest were either impossible, needed careful negotiation or sheer brute force.

And at home it meant almost every day I could move around. There were some days when my arms/hands were too tired to operate the controls but mostly I could get around. Wow, freedom! Although, as my children will attest, it took many weeks to perfect my navigation and unfortunately for them many run over toes and screams of pain on their part to get the speed thing sorted. I was a speed demon. After months of not being able to move faster than the person pushing me, I was off and nothing was stopping me.

What Am I Going To Do Now

JANUARY – MARCH 2007

In January 2007, we had a camping holiday at the beach. I couldn't take my power chair due to space in the car and sand getting into the motor, so I had to go back to the manual chair and my sticks. I had improved a little bit so I could walk with my sticks for short distances and we camped in front of the toilet block.

It was beautiful to be by the sea and although I couldn't go in the ocean, I could get onto the beach and feel the sand between my toes. It was the most carefree I had felt for a long time.

I love the freedom of sleeping in a tent and eating from a barbeque, and with my chair I always had a seat! With Matthew to share the care of the children and the meal preparation, I could have a rest. I felt positive.

When we returned to Braidwood I returned to acupuncture in Canberra, thanks to the kindness of my friend who continued to drive me once or twice a week. My digestion had improved but I felt like my progress was stagnating.

I could walk short distances with my sticks or walker, with my right leg dragging and sometimes needing to give it a kick start. I was being showered every day, and had assistance to prepare food and do my domestics. For any distances both my arms and my legs would get too tired to use any walking aids and so I needed the chair. And there were still many days when I just needed the chair.

I was beginning to accept this was my life and began to think about my future, again.

I still had a handful of students and had now finished the website, but teaching was becoming more difficult with the deterioration of cognitive function, and the thought of taking another writing job was not enticing.

So what else could I do?

Errant cells

At the same time I had an inkling to get a pap smear. I hadn't had one for a while and something didn't feel quite right. Sure enough the results came back positive with middle grade cell change. An appointment was made to have a colposcopy (a glorified pap smear with a gynaecologist) at Canberra Hospital.

The photograph of my cervix showed a large mass

of precancerous cells spread around the surface. With such a large surface area of cells to remove, it was decided to do it under general in case my cervix began haemorrhaging. I would be notified about the date.

Thank god for my inkling. As frightening as this was, I had probably made it in time. Of course, the whole procedure exhausted me and I needed help to get dressed and back into my chair. The strangest thing was that I wasn't particularly surprised; I think I was getting used to bad news that wasn't as bad as it could be. Perhaps my guardian angel was still with me.

A date was made for the surgery and I booked transport for day procedure to burn off the errant cells under general. It was months away so it went to the back of my mind to give that under-layer of anxiety of not quite here but threatening; like thunderclouds in the distance when the washing isn't quite dry.

The Fulcrum
Meditation Retreat

MARCH 2007

We all have moments in our lives that feel like fulcrums of destiny; a point on which your life rests and the choice you make will determine your future direction.

The Dru Meditation weekend was such a moment.

I had been to an afternoon of Dru Yoga with my old yoga teacher and there were flyers for a weekend of meditation in Canberra. Something in my mind just clicked, "I want to go to that". The logistics of getting to Canberra for the weekend, in a wheelchair didn't occur to me, I just knew I wanted to go.

So I talked to my husband and he was supportive – I think at that stage he was ready to try anything. He believed in the spiritual/emotional/psychological basis of illness before we even met and had watched me heal asthma at a weekend meditation retreat. He had also watched me work my way back to walking in Britain.

I think he was hoping for a miracle. I am so lucky he had faith in me (either that or he was desperate, either way it was all good).

I filled out my little form and sent in my cheque before I could think about it…it was only after that I started to think about how.

My old friend, the saboteur, was close by as the weekend got closer and I had not done anything to organise getting there. It never ceases to amaze me how strong one's saboteur can be when you want to drag yourself out a hole.

"Maybe I won't go; maybe it was a stupid idea." Then out of nowhere, "Maybe I'll ring the Dru office". There was a feeling of battle between the forces of good and evil in my mind or maybe it was the forces of higher self and ego.

The same dulcet tones, again – how lucky am I? I explained my situation and she was so supportive and kind and generous, as she is. There should be a word that means all those things and it would be this woman's name, and then I could just say her name and everyone would know exactly what I meant. Suffice it to say this woman is the embodiment of grace.

"Let me see what I can do and I'll get back to you".

The first arrangement was to stay with a long time Dru teacher, who was assisting at the workshop. Then when this person realised I was disabled and her house would therefore be unsuitable, a room at the hotel venue of retreat was booked – at her expense. Once again I found myself in tears at someone's kindness and generosity.

In my time in the Dru community since that weekend, I have realised this kind of generosity is not unusual – no one ever has to do anything in solitude – and yet I feel this particular gesture may well have contributed to the turning of the tide that has forever changed my life, and I will feel eternal gratitude to her for her kindness.

This seemed to tip the balance and I soon was able to arrange transport to and from the venue with Anglicare. It was sorted, I was going – help!

The first day was great. I loved being back in that particular Dru environment – warm, fun and supportive. I meditated, managed a little visualisation and was even able to do some physical postures. But the toilets were on the other side of the room and so I didn't drink a lot of water to avoid wheeling across to go to the toilet. I drank in the evening but perhaps the damage had been done or maybe I simply did too much physical work.

Whatever it was, I woke in the morning with the mother of all headaches. I felt nauseous, my vision was disturbed and I felt dysfunction and/or pain in every part of my body. Nonetheless, I confided in my benefactor that I had been considering applying for the yoga teacher training course.

I felt vaguely stupid (not to mention a little embarrassed) thinking about a yoga teacher training course from the glorious vantage point of a motorised wheelchair but I couldn't stop thinking about it. I couldn't believe her enthusiasm for my idea.

I decided to stay and have a rest while she went to the beginning of the session but the pain was too severe to sleep and thoughts were doing the circuit in my mind. "Could I?"

"No, of course, not"

"But maybe…"

Eventually I gave up and went to the session. The pain and dysfunction had become so severe I couldn't even lift a glass to my mouth without spilling, so I just sat. I visualised or meditated.

Then without noticing the exact moment of ascension, I found myself in the most extraordinary peace. Time had stopped and I was seeing the world from a deeper place; a softer, lighter place where the physical realities of my life were far less important than this inner serenity.

Once again I had dropped into this state of mind where I could hold excruciating pain and beauty in one hand, through stillness. So I sat in this room with 50 or so other people, in the centre of light, while pain and other neurological sensations swirled around me like a rampaging tornado. "Let it rampage, I will sit in the eye of the storm."

"If only I could live like this … maybe I can … the yoga teacher training course. Maybe I can learn how to share this with other disabled people, maybe I can teach teenagers … maybe it's time to learn to live like this."

Both the female tutors were very encouraging. "If you can't do the postures, you can always visualise, and it can be more powerful." Such warmth!

So I booked a mentoring session with the senior tutor, Andrew again. I tried very hard to hide just how mad I actually was but I felt I couldn't hide anything – bugger! There are very few things I remember from this weekend but the warmth in his eyes during that session I will never forget.

It *was* time I learnt to live life in this peace and I *could* teach other disabled people how to find this peace. Oh my god, a decision?

A yoga teacher in a wheelchair – huh, I really am mad!!!

The Path to the Module

MARCH–MAY 2007

On the way home from the meditation weekend I talked to the respite carer about my experiences and my ambitions to become yoga teacher and she was so supportive; I was blown away. Perhaps she was as mad as I was.

I now had carers for bathing (I was prone to falling, toppling over and losing the use of my mind and body while showering, forget getting out and dressing – this took some time to recover); carers for peeling and preparing vegetables; carers for domestic duties; and respite carers. It was a revolving door, and carers and health professionals alike would shout as they came in.

In addition to the carers, there was a physiotherapist who visited me as often as her schedule permitted, a psychologist who visited for a consultation once a month, community nurses, care coordinators and case officers.

They were often the only people other than family I saw and talked with so they became my confidantes; some have become friends long after the need for care has passed. I was so lucky to receive such care and kindness.

They were unanimous in their support for my ideas of training to be a yoga teacher. Could be they were all mad as well.

Applying was painfully prolonged due to procrastination; fear overcame the process more times than I can count. And I really thought it was completely mad to even think about doing it. Anyway, I did and even stranger, I was accepted.

They really must have been mad too.

The errant cells were also in the back of my mind and came to the surface regularly but almost as a separate track. Perhaps at the time I had several separate tracks that ran parallel but independently of each other, crossing or joining only at rare junction points.

This could be why it took me so long to realise the surgery was scheduled two days after the module finished; or to organise the child care for Nicola, transport and accommodation for the module or indeed transport for the surgery.

(Dru yoga teacher training was organised in nine four-day modules over three years beginning at the end of May 2007.)

There was the unreality and procrastination aspect of the teacher training. I think there was part of me that didn't tell the rest of me I was actually going to do the teacher training. I have operated a lot like this in the past. I am not quite sure of the rationale but procrastinating full disclosure with myself also delayed disclosure with the rest of the world and consequently the organisation of details. Repeatedly I have realised the extra anxiety this has caused, the futility of delaying and the inconvenience I have caused other people by my inability to simply be straight, and this was no different.

The junction of all the divergent trains of thought became apparent only a couple of weeks before the module.

Module 1

MAY – JUNE 2007

What was so special about the module to begin such a deep transformation? I have asked myself many times since. And, you know, I wonder if it was the hospital experience immediately after that sealed my direction.

The module was four days of learning the basics of Dru Yoga postures, sequences and principles. There was very little I could do physically but I watched, listened and visualised, only half believing it was going to impact on me personally.

I opened myself completely to the teaching so I could learn as much as possible. Every mode of learning was operating because I couldn't write to take notes. I created a movie in which I was the camera and the actor and the stage. I still remember words and sensations from that first module. (**How to visualise** p.133)

I felt stronger each day. How blessed I was to be

there. My accommodation had been sponsored by Anglicare so I was able to motor down to my room each evening, motor into the bathroom, right to the shower or toilet, and relax. I felt so cumbersome but no one else seemed to notice and the whole Dru community seemed to embrace this strange idea of a person in a wheelchair at yoga teacher training.

Yet despite the physical disability, the process seemed to come so naturally. Meditation in motion (without the motion, for me), for four days. It all just seemed to click. Another mentoring session showed me that my view of myself was already changing in the positive.

When Matthew came to pick me up at the end of the four days he said I was the best he had seen me in a couple of years! It was certainly a powerful experience, but without the events of the following week could have stayed just a nice experience, so I am very grateful for what came next.

Two days after the module, I was scheduled for a minor procedure to remove pre-cancerous cells from my cervix under a general anaesthetic. The procedure was straightforward and successful but I woke from the anaesthetic unable to move my bits, breathe properly or swallow. I didn't know when my bladder was full and couldn't speak properly.

There was confusion and fear in the people around me but still carrying the effects of four days of meditation, I felt detached. I began to practice the relaxation skills I had just spent four days learning.

The more I practiced, the more I noticed how fear impedes decision making and functioning, and so the more I practiced.

I also began visualising the practices and sequences we had just learned: Energy Block Release 1 (**EBR1** p.133), the dog, the cat and the beautiful flowing tree (founding sequences and postues of Dru Yoga). I didn't want to lose contact with the practices and, well, I didn't have anything else to do. My mind was the only part that was active.

It was amazing. I had never really understood the phrase, "I am not my body, I am not my emotions, am not my mind", until then. My body was motionless but I could feel the energy move through my body as I visualised moving from one posture to another. My emotions were on the brink of fear yet constant relaxations and yoga kept the fear flowing and on the periphery; creating distance from the panic. And although my mind was confused with this MS exacerbation, something higher was operating to enable clarity and depth in my yoga practice.

When I was visualising I could remember tones of voices, see the teachers demonstrating, smell the smells, and feel the feelings in my body as I imagined doing yoga. My mind became clear and smooth. When I was not visualising I felt the classic MS fogginess.

Within four days I was ready to go home and continue my journey into my mind. As a result of the surgery, I had lost all the ground I had gained at the module but now there was something I could do in my armchair, wheelchair, lying awake in the middle of the night and while my daughter watched 'ABC Kids'. And I did – all day, every day.

These practices are part of me now in a way I never thought was possible. My body seems to breathe them in.

As my physical condition improved, gradually (I had now stopped Chinese medicine so any improvement was due to yoga) I was able to do more physical postures but visualisation was still the bulk of my practice.

I fitted my physical and mental practice into my life in small bits throughout the day: with kids, while I was doing stuff, while teaching. Basically in and around the rest of my life, even at night.

As a chronic insomniac I had spent many hours tossing and turning in bed between my daughter and my husband. Now, I mentally practiced yoga. I don't think I got any more sleep during this period but I was certainly a lot more relaxed and peaceful, waking in the morning after doing an hour or two of yoga through the night.

Doing my practice in this way enabled me to get intimately connected to the postures and sequences, using my breath to deepen the postures and my awareness, and begin to sense the energy flow.

And of course all of this inner growth was transforming my relationship with the world as relationships on all levels became easier and calmer. (see ***The practice*** p.135)

With the increased body awareness and concentration I could imagine energy from the breath flowing through the actual muscles to move them, mentally and/or physically. I was visualising yoga practices from the inside of my body.

I felt like I inhabited the postures in a way I had never done. I also felt like I was beginning to inhabit myself again.

How to visualise

Visualising came in three stages
- *First I would watch the demonstration and listen carefully to the words.*
- *Then I would feel the movements in my body, like I was doing the same movements the demonstrators were doing.*
- *Lastly, I would close my eyes and imagine myself doing the movements as they were described.*

Energy Block Release 1

The Energy Block Release (EBR) sequences are a series of Dru practices but the concept of moving energy around the body using a sequence of movements and visualisations is an ancient one. See martial arts such as tai chi, qi gong and other yoga traditions. The reason the concept has survived through traditions, revolutions and thousands upon thousands of practitioners over centuries is simple – it works, on every level of the body-mind-spirit complex.

A balanced sequence of movements, stretching and soothing the body-mind-spirit system, is easy to remember while encapsulating the essence of the tradition. It is not only relatively easy to learn but relatively easy to teach and practice, maintaining integrity of the tradition.

In Dru the focus is to use Energy Block Release (EBR) sequences to remove blocks from our energy system so energy that was once trapped can become available to us. This energy can then be directed to particular parts of the body with specific asanas or other sequences.

You see, what I've learnt from my practice is that everything the body does is sending messages to your mind and everything your mind does is sending messages to your body and spirit. The mind, body and spirit are in constant interaction.

In a balanced and integrated system, this interaction is harmonic, producing a beautiful composition called wellbeing, which I've also discovered doesn't necessarily mean injury or disability free. We have all heard of people with permanent disability, chronic illness or sometimes even terminal illness who radiate wellness; and I have even experienced it myself. It simply means, within the constraints of their physical condition, that person has found harmony and balance.

Energy Block Release 1(EBR1) is the foundation EBR in Dru and is a sequence of movements that works through the whole body while opening the heart then moving stuck energy from the base of the spine into an open heart.

It is in itself, a complete practice.

The practice

When I returned home, having begun visualising in hospital, I continued in the way I had begun. The main practices I remember focusing on at the time were the Foundation Relaxation, Energy Block Release 1 and Marjariasana (the Cat, all practices I still do now, both in my mind and physically).

There were some points I discovered along the way that were vital to my practice and I want to share them with you because so many people find visualising intimidating, and just as many people find establishing a regular practice similarly intimidating.

These ideas have worked so beautifully for me with Dru Yoga and meditation, but I think they would work with any modality.

- *Short and often*
- *So that's how it feels to relax*

- *Do something every day*
- *If you stop in the middle of a sequence, just start again when you can*
- *If you can't visualise it, don't do it*
- *Work with instinct*

Let's take each of them, one at a time.

Short and often

This discovery, like all of the others, was an accident that arose out of necessity rather than genius-inspired creativity.

Since the spiral towards physical breakdown in 2004, my stamina had been compromised, to say the least, so I began doing something I have never done before – practice every day.

I found that even the limited exercises I had been given by physiotherapists and my own random yoga postures resulted in slight MS exacerbations when done all at once. When the speech therapy and the occupational therapy is added, it all seemed too overwhelming to contemplate.

The answer for me was to break it all up into bits and do them through the day. That makes it sound far more considered than it was. I wanted to walk and I wanted use my hands and I wanted to speak and swallow, and so I wanted to do it all, and the only way I could was to do it in bits all through the day. I was practicing all day in bits.

I was always stretching or exercising my

hands, rotating my ankles, massaging my hands or feet; becoming aware of my swallowing and speech. Whereas before I found it difficult to do anything two days in a row, now I was doing stuff every day, all day.

I was becoming aware of my body. I knew my condition was improving and I knew I was regaining some sense of control over a life that had spiralled out of control.

What I didn't know was that I was laying the foundations for a daily practice that later enabled me to walk when I had accepted life in a wheelchair. I continue to practice like this now, always doing something, no matter how small.

The advantages of a practice done short and often are:
- *It's not intimidating because you don't feel like you have to find a huge tract of time to fit in your practice;*
- *It reduces fatigue associated with longer practices;*
- *Because you're doing your practice all through the day, your body is constantly being warmed and your energy system lubricated;*
- *This works emotionally and spiritually as well; and*
- *Finally, and perhaps most importantly, practicing in this way gives you the opportunity to integrate your practice into your daily life.*

So that's how it feels to relax!

I remember the moment I first knew what it felt like to relax.

Before I started classes I had no idea what people meant when they said "relax". I didn't know how to do it and I didn't know what it felt like. The first time I had any sense of what relaxation might feel like was in a yoga class – "Aaah, so that's what it feels like".

That was the beginning. Since then I have deepened my experience and practice of relaxation, but it hasn't always been easy, and sometimes a downright struggle. I had spent my life as a wound up spring and even though I had been given the key to unwind, my body and mind seemed reluctant to let go; like a Jack-in-the-box that didn't want to come out when the box was opened.

Even now I sometimes have to be reminded of the value of a practice that has saved my bacon so many times.

It is possible. I have learned to scan my body in any situation, find where I am holding tension and let it go. It is possible to become aware in a bank queue of a thumb making a whole hand tight or toes gripping on to the earth in a yoga posture or neck and shoulders carrying the weight of the world while cooking dinner. It is possible to do a whole body relaxation in a few moments, on a hospital bed, having a glorified pap smear or my legs waxed, or in my first job interview in years.

All this is possible, I know, because I have done it, and if I can you can ... but you have to practice. There are no shortcuts.

The importance of relaxation in a healing body or a chronically ill body or, in fact, any body at all cannot be understated. If your body and mind are always in a state of alert the resulting cascade of chemical production is highly toxic to the functioning of your mind body, in every respect.

The fight or flight response is designed to be exactly that: a short lived response to a crisis, and after the crisis is over the body flushes the toxic chemicals and returns to normal. However, ongoing stress puts the body into the flight or flight response permanently, reducing our ability to make good decisions, be creative and most importantly, be present.

Many prevalent chronic illnesses, such as hypertension, high blood pressure, heart disease and depression, have stress as a key risk factor. MS deterioration and exacerbations are also strongly linked to stress.

And it seems that being relaxed through the day is not enough; the optimum practice is to thoroughly relax yourself as often as you can, ideally at least once a day.

So learn a relaxation practice and practice it ... regularly.

Do something every day

This may not sound like rocket science but to me it was. Many intellectual, sporting and creative pursuits have stressed the importance of practicing daily rather than once or twice a week but it had been lost on me; yoga and meditation is no different.

When you first begin, find something that resonates with you and do it. It needs to be a practice that feels right for you and your body because you won't remember to do it unless it means something to you.

Through the text of this book I will include many of the practices that got me started and kept me going through the most difficult times of my journey.

If you stop in the middle of a sequence, just start again when you remember

This is another really important point, partly because I used to do a lot of visualising in the middle of the night, and partly because serious fatigue affects your concentration, and partly because sometimes life just gets in the way.

When I began the yoga teacher training course, I was an insomniac but instead of tossing and turning, mentally going down a spiral into despair, I began visualising yoga. And frequently I would drift off into sleep in the middle of a sequence (most commonly, EBR 1) and just as *frequently I would wake with the movement I had fallen asleep with on my mind*

At first, I got annoyed with myself for falling asleep (how is that for self-abuse – telling myself off for falling asleep in the middle of the night?!) then I started to realise I was waking in the morning feeling like I had just come out of a yoga class. So instead of getting annoyed when I fell asleep, I just picked up from where I fell asleep.

Interruption would often happen through the day as well.

"If I can pick it up from sleep, I can pick it up in my day as well".

From then on it didn't bother me if Nicola interrupted a practice or if a carer or other health-care professional arrived in the middle a practice or even if I lost concentration – my mind just took me right back to where I stopped.

This opened up a whole new field of practice for me. It meant I could practice mentally anywhere, anytime, and if I was interrupted, I just continued on when I could. This was essential for someone who had their practice room and meditation shrine in the family lounge room.

Sequences like the Energy Block Release sequences, Salute to the Sun and relaxation practices can be quite difficult to practice in one go, particularly with the cognitive and fatigue issues of MS and other chronic illnesses, wheth-

er you are doing it physically or visualising, but
don't worry – your mind -body will remember
and pick up where you left off.
This same principle works for relaxation and meditation.

If you can't visualise it, don't do it

When I was visualising the Cat and the spinal
wave in EBR 1 a lot between Module 1 and 2,
I was trying really hard to move each vertebra,
one at a time, 'like the cogs in a bike chain' or
'the pearls in a necklace'. I just couldn't get
particular vertebra to move separately and I
found myself getting really frustrated. I wanted
to be the perfect yogi with a clear spine.

My teacher simply said my energy system
wasn't ready to release the blocks between the
vertebras and I didn't need to force it. So easy.

I stopped and began to recognise other places
in my visualising practice I couldn't go or places
in sequences I stopped, and when I could push
through it and when I couldn't.

I learnt (am still learning) it's not about
being the external, idealised perfect yogi; it's
about being the perfect me – working with the
mind/body/spirit I have now. Accepting who I
am in this moment, with all my physical/mental
and emotional imperfections is being the perfect
yogi. I cannot be the master of anyone else's body;
I can only be the master of my own.

For me this also answers many questions
about contra-indications and visualisation: when

the contraindication or inability to do a practice is due to a physical injury or limitation (recent surgery or physical disability, for example), try visualising, gently.

However, if the reason behind the contraindication is energetic (for example, certain postures are contraindicated during the first three days of menstruation), then the best policy is to avoid the posture altogether (this may also be the case for abdominal surgery and postures that stir up the energy in that area of the body).

The principle that has worked for me is: if a posture is designed to stimulate an area of the body/energy system you want to remain calm (e.g. the lower abdominal area after surgery), then don't do it – physically or mentally.

Another example from my own practice is inverted or upside down postures and severe headaches or brain conditions. When the cognitive symptoms of MS hit, I can feel ridiculously fuzzy, slow, depressed, detached (not in a Zen way), have brain-freeze, sometimes go bi-polar and experience the most debilitating headaches.

There are times I can't even think about going upside down and others when my head cannot even go below my heart. There is no discussion, no negotiation with myself, I just can't do it. Horizontal is as close as I can get.

So be sensitive to yourself, and if you can't

visualise a posture or sequence, maybe you're not supposed to be doing it; and if you're at all unsure, err on the side of caution and follow the physical contra-indications.

Work with instinct

The thing about a personal practice is that it is a personal practice. Yes, there are guidelines and safety issues; some practices that go well together and others that don't, but there is no 'one-size-fits-all' programme for wellbeing. The secret, if there is one, is to find the practices that suit your mind and body and life.

We don't grow up with much faith in our own judgement in our culture, and a chronic illness that's such a mystery and so unpredictable, like MS, destroys what threads of faith that have managed to hold on. Growing my own practice in the way I continue to do has given me a more intimate relationship with myself than I have ever experienced in my life, even before MS.

So listen to your body and become your own best friend.

Building a personal practice

The essence of building a daily personal practice is to find the cracks in your day and insert a practice, any practice no matter how small. Then without even noticing, the cracks get bigger and so do the practices and before you know it you have a personal practice. Be grateful for what you can do, and what you can do will expand.

Module 2

SEPTEMBER 2007

My state of mind had been steadily improving as I got closer to the module, until I came against the struggle with my saboteur to actually get there – "No money, can't get there, I don't deserve the funding ..."

In the weeks before the module I also began to feel scattered and frustrated, and began to look a little strung out. Matthew asked if perhaps I was doing too much yoga, so I slowed down a little and by the time the module arrived I was a little calmer.

Somehow I overcame my inner opposition and found my way there.

When I arrived in my wheelchair at the second module, I felt incredibly unprepared.

"All of the other students would have been doing the physical practices for the last four months and I have just been thinking about it".

The first thing we did after activation was to split into small groups to discuss our practice during the time since the last module. My heart sank. "What can I possibly say about my practice?" speaking openly about my personal experience has always been difficult because I felt my experience was either wrong or boring or both and the listener(s) would judge me as a fraud or boring or wrong.

I was the last to speak, and I listened as one by one my peers detailed their practices and their experiences and their emotions, and my heart sank further with each one.

"What do I say?"

My turn.

"I have been visualising, a lot. I have been getting stronger, I think, I have been getting calmer, I think." I'm screaming on the inside.

The group asked me if there was anything they could do to help. I was so surprised they would want to help and all I could think was to ask them for notes because I still wasn't writing. Then they asked if they could help me physically with postures.

Oh my goodness, no, and for a moment forgot about my insecurities.

"When I get to a point when I can't do it physically, I see the energy moving inside my body and let the energy do it." And I showed them with one of the movements from EBR1.

"On my own I can only raise my arm halfway but when I close my eyes and see the energy and allow my mind to do it, my arm raises all the way, almost on its own."

I had been aware of the expression on Trish's face (Trish was one of the senior tutors and one of the original teachers to say I could visualise) changing as I was speaking and now it was almost shock. Immediately I thought I'd said something wrong and wished I hadn't started talking. I wished I hadn't forgotten I was wrong.

Trish very quietly said that was quite an advanced practice. Even still, I felt wrong. Later in the module one of the graduate helpers said "I hear you've doing some amazing things with visualising". How did she hear that? What amazing things?

I was still thinking I was wrong. It has taken 2½ years and a shirt-load more practice to realise I wasn't wrong.

The next thing that happened was again in small groups, smaller groups of about four or five this time. We were reviewing EBR1, teaching it to each other. An amazing thing happened during that session: I found that with all the visualising I had done, I could do the whole practice, physically.

Not only could I do it but I could do it well and teach others how to do it. I had spent so many hours visualising my spine moving one vertebra at a time that I could get much closer to doing it than my peers and I could show them. How bizarre!

As the module continued, my confidence grew and I tried more and more physical yoga. Of course, I was very tired and sometimes too tired to even visualise but the seeds had been sown for a physicality I had never expected to return to.

The thing I have wondered about is muscle tone. When I was being fitted for a leg brace during the winter of 2007, I hardly had enough strength in my quads (muscles at the front of the thigh) to lift my leg off the ground. Yet during module 2 I could do some physical yoga.

How can that be?

I still don't really understand but as I have been writing these chapters it has occurred to me that perhaps it was also due to visualisation. If the same part of the brain is stimulated when we imagine as when we experience the actual action, couldn't we also be building musculature as we practice?

On the second day of the module I experienced something I have always struggled with through my life – the feeling of alienation from the people around me. The same old feelings of judgement and feeling judged; not being liked. I have never expected to be liked (in fact, quite the opposite) and have never expected to fit in to groups, but I wanted this to be different.

So, when I went back to my room I opened the Gita with the question in my mind. The answer was to offer myself and so the next day I did, and the difference in how I felt was astonishing. I had done this with Matthew but hadn't been able to in the rest of my life. Now I tried to see the best in people, and it worked.

Every module during the course I offered myself to the people I felt the most judged by or the most judgemental of and it changed the way I related to people all through my life. I found some of my closest friends in the process.

So, in the spirit of giving on the third day, I seized an opportunity to teach my peers visualisation. This was so unlike me and not something I would ever have done before the module. The small group I was with were too tired to undergo the teaching practice we were supposed to be doing so I offered to take them through a visualisation of EBR1.

It was amazing to be taking my friends through what for me had become like breathing. It was like living inside-out. And for me, who always lived very inside-inside, it was confronting and affirming at the same time, and possibly another one of those moments that changed my future a little. They loved it and it deepened the way they found the practice afterwards. So, it's not just me then.

Then, on the final day came a moment in med-itation when I reached out to another student who was struggling to remain in stillness. From within my meditation I felt her struggle but didn't know what I should do.

To be honest I thought twice about helping because I was in such a lovely space myself. "What can I do, anyway?" But then I remembered the verse in the Gita and reached out to her in my mind, to support her. Her struggle seemed to ease, and after the meditation I turned to her and held her as she cried. "How did you know?" she asked.

I don't know how I knew, I just did.

There has been a special bond between us since that day and a little later, between modules, I reached out to her again in my mind. When we met up at the next module we discovered it was the same time she landed with meditation.

It was a little 'ooby-gooby', but testament to the oneness of life and how we can support each other through the difficulties of life, just with our mind.

At another mentoring session with Andrew it was amazing it was to see how far I'd come in such a short time. Andrew asked me about how I saw my prana. I had no idea what he was talking about. Then he said, "Mine is a river of gold". That's it!

That's what I've been seeing move through my body, the energy that has been helping me do yoga postures; what I had tried to describe in the small group at the beginning of the module. So, now I have a river of gold of prana – awesome!

Andrew suggested I use the river of gold in yoga but maybe I can use my river of gold not just in my yoga but also the rest of my life? I had been getting stronger day by day through the module so why not use it at home, to walk and chop carrots and…

What Happened Next?

SEPTEMBER – NOVEMBER 2007

I have been procrastinating writing this part of my journey; partly because I hardly believe it myself and partly because I want to accurately describe what I experienced during this period. However, I can procrastinate no longer and so I am just going to sit with this until I have written through the next two months of my journey.

I had stopped going to acupuncture before Module 1 but was still boiling the herbs for my digestion then, midway to module 2, I even stopped the herbs. They had worked so well for my digestion and fatigue but it became too difficult to continue getting them from Canberra, and my instinct was to stop.

So now any improvement in my condition was due to yoga and meditation.

Silverchair and Powderfinger

Silverchair and Powderfinger are two of my favourite Australian bands and when Gabriel told me they were playing together in Canberra, we agreed it was a must see concert and bought tickets.

Before I decided to be a yoga teacher.

As the date got closer, I realised the concert was two days after the second module. I contemplated not going, angsted over getting more respite support and fought with my son over whether his friend could travel with us but finally it was sorted. We were going; with carer and the wheelchair van, meeting the friend in Canberra.

So, two days after the module one of my favourite carers arrived to pick us up in the big blue van and take us to Canberra. I have never been to a concert in a wheelchair and I was a little concerned about how it would go.

All the way into Canberra, Gabe talked with the carer while I sat in my chair, locked into the back of the van, contemplating and visualising what I had learned in the module. By the time I arrived at the concert I was established in an altered state of consciousness and open to whatever was about to happen.

We met up with Gabe's friend and found there was a crip- ple platform – raised and right behind the mixing desk. Awe- some! I was allowed only one carer so I sent both teenagers into the crowd and I settled in for meditation and visualisation.

I have always been intimidated by humanity en-masse (well, humanity at all, to be honest),and tended to avoid large gatherings or been quite fearful for the entire time I was amongst them, but this time, after my experiences at the module, I was intrigued and my heart was open.

While I waited for the concert to begin I practiced EBR2 in my mind. I still love the balance between heart opening and physicality in EBR2, and then it was a revelation. Even visualising the heaven and earth stretch, dynamic squats, sitting forward bend and the cobra gave my body a feeling of spacious, energised calm.

I alternated this with Deep Yogic Breath (**Deep yogic breath** below) and the feeling in my mind was spacious stillness and joy. At the same time the wooden platform throbbed with the bass drum and the throb travelled all the way up the whole chair to connect with my body just behind my heart.

So for three hours I meditated and yoga-ed and listened to the awesome tunes of the support band, Powderfinger and Silverchair, and possibly for the first time in my life felt part of the human race.

Thank god for yoga, thank god for respite and thank god for my children. I am alive!

Deep Yogic Breath (DYB)

Caution:
- *Changing your breathing cycle can be a powerful practice so be aware of the feelings in your mind and body;*

- *If you begin to feel any unpleasant sensations, such as tingles, light-headedness or giddiness return to normal breathing, lie down on your stomach or go and so something soothing and relaxing – ALWAYS LISTEN TO THE LIMITS OF YOUR OWN BODY; and*
- *If you have a heart condition or blood pressure issues, don't breathe too deeply and don't hold the breath.*
- *DYB uses every part of the lungs in each breath.*
- *Begin with a few breaths into the lower part of your lungs using your diaphragm to expand the lungs. Repeat this for a few breaths.*
- *Focus on the middle part of your lungs around your heart and take a few breaths. This is also called 'thoracic breath'.*
- *Then raise your awareness up into top part of your lungs, either side of your collarbones. Repeat for a few breaths.*
- *In one breath, breathe from your diaphragm to your collarbones, pause and breathe out, using your diaphragm to exhale the breath from the base to the top of your lungs.*

Walking to the Beat of My Heart

The day after the concert I felt amazing. It was like energy was charging through my system. The friend who had been driving me to the acupuncturist in Canberra visited. She said I was the best she had ever seen me but was experiencing severe neck pain herself.

I looked at her neck and saw the area around C7 was red and swollen. I put my hand over the area and left it there for a while. She said my hand was hot, almost unbearably hot.

An incredible stillness surrounded us as we sat out in the sun behind my house. My friend's neck pain eased, enabling her to drive home and she went straight to bed and slept. When I spoke to her that afternoon, the pain in her neck had eased significantly and a week later it was still relatively pain free.

But the following day brought the post-module

hangover. It was something I was to get used to over the two and a half years of the course. We spend four days in a loving, supportive environment, all experiencing 'stuff' as the yoga, relaxation and meditation releases years of stuck emotion. As a consequence, the friendships we form are based on surprising intimacy and honesty; all talking the same language.

Then we come home (and I frequently felt half-baked, like I didn't quite complete whatever process I was in) to the lives we have constructed; children who need their parent back NOW, partners, friends and work colleagues, none of whom have been through the same transformative process we have. Yet somehow we have to fit back in, like putting on your favourite clothes but your body shape has changed and they don't fit so well.

I think I always felt a little grief and a little guilt. I felt grief for leaving what seemed like an oasis of relating, with all its associated difficulties, and because I didn't have it at home; and guilt because I felt grief.

Added to the emotional issues was the energetic hangover. We spend four days doing strong postures and meditation techniques, from 9am until 6pm, and while I was still visualising at least 50% of the time, I was still moving energy around my body. I always feel it takes a few days for all that energy to come to its new equilibrium.

After landing from the Dru orbit I did snuggle back in to my life in Braidwood and began to ask myself what to do with the information I had gained from the module.

After a short time of treading water I began my practice again.

During my mentoring with Andrew he had suggested I start listening to Chakra Dharanam recordings by Chris Barrington, one of the founders of Dru Worldwide. I hadn't really thought about actually doing it because I had no extra money for buying resources but on the last day of the module I discovered the discount basket with discontinued cassettes and there were the last copies of the Chakra Dharanam I and II. $5 each – bargain!

I added them to my daily practice. Every night I read Nicola a story and sat with her while she went to sleep. I had been in the habit of going to sleep with her as her bed was next to mine and I was usually exhausted by then anyway. The only difference now was I put my headphones on and listened to the dulcet tones of Chris.

At first I found myself getting annoyed with his mannerisms and arguing with him in my mind but I kept listening, partly because Andrew had recommended it and partly because I knew there was something there for me, if only I could get past the personality. Besides, each time I listened I felt this extraordinary sense of peace which got deeper each time I listened.

I have been racking my brains and reading through my journal to find the switch but I can't find the specific moment or thought. All I can find is a building momentum, an indescribable burning desire to walk, leftover from the module. This was combined with an inner knowing (God knows where from) that I could use my 'yoga energy'; my river of gold.

Regardless of where it came from, one day in late September, I took my wheelie walker (and my daughter) and walked out the front door. Walking is perhaps an exaggeration; it was more a glorified shuffle, relying heavily on the walker. We had ramps for the wheelchair so I tentatively walked the walker down the ramps, to the front gate and out!

For the second time in twelve months, I understood freedom. The grass looked greener, the sky looked bluer; to sound clichéd, everything looked brighter, bolder and bigger.

I turned left and 'walked' down to the corner. Every step was an exercise in concentration as I put the heel down and then the middle and then the ball, and finally my toes. Each step was like this, with Nicola beside me asking questions the whole way.

"Where are we going mummy?"

"Why don't we have the wheelchair, mummy?"

"Why are we going so slowly, mummy?" etc, etc, etc

I don't know how many questions can be asked in a short period of time but I'm sure she came close to some uncelebrated record.

I was absolutely present in every movement. I so don't know where this came from. The feeling I have now when I remember that first 'walk' was that there was a strength that came from beneath the base of my spine and rose up through the core of my being.

When I got to the corner I had to stop because I couldn't move. My core stability muscles were about to collapse as were my leg and arms. I slowed down my breathing and imagined my river of gold flowing into my arms then into my core and finally down my legs. And most importantly, I think now, I relaxed; stopped trying to hold on. This is what I call 'realigning my energy'.

I knew to do this because it worked in module. So I waited until I was ready to go back. Slowly, slowly (More questions from Nicola).

The return trip was even slower and more conscious than the outgoing journey, all to the commentary of my very supportive four year-old-daughter.

This walk to the corner and back marks the beginning of my physical recovery. As I write it now, I realise it was also the beginning of my journey into presence. Every skill I regained, every sensation I recovered was accompanied by this same technique: *slowly, breathe, become aware of energy flow, presence in the moment*; and this was all made possible by the hours I spent visualising the energy flow through my body while I imagined yoga.

Most of the rest of my life had been played out reliving the past or fantasising about the future but for once I was absolutely in the present; rejoicing in every step and not thinking about the next one.

When I arrived home I was completely exhausted and collapsed on my cripple armchair. Nicola climbed up on my lap and cuddled in. Somehow she knew the significance of what had just happened, and was very quiet and still.

I was unable to go out again for a few days but continued to read and visualise the postures and sequences from module 2, occasionally doing some physical yoga.

Again, I heard the silent command to try again. This time I crossed the road and travelled a few metres further on. Wow! My soul leapt for joy. Again I had to stop and realign my energy but I did it and Nicola was with my every step.

Back again to the comfort of my cripple chair to rest for another few days.

At this stage I was concentrating on walking because as the MS seemed to have been retreating from my legs, it was getting worse in my arms and hands. They ached constantly and my fine motor co-ordination was *so* not good. I was regaining independence in one aspect and simultaneously losing it in another.

I now used wrist splints on both arms, particularly while on the keyboard, to keep my hands in an ergonomically neutral position, thereby reducing the energy required to keep the hands working. The payoff though was even more reduced fine motor co-ordination. For example, my writing became illegible, signature unrecognisable and carrots were cut chunky.

I was so grateful, not for the first time, that someone had the foresight to fund my Dragon. Now when I couldn't use my hands I could use my Dragon, and when my speech went I went back to the keyboard.

Balancing between hands and speech meant I could still write my portfolios for the course and emails to keep in contact.

(NB: during the yoga teacher training course, students have to write portfolios on each technique we learn, outlining alignment points, contra-indications, modifications, difficulties, alternatives and how the posture/ sequence makes us feel)

It was, in fact, in writing the portfolios for this module that I discovered another potential use and benefit of visualisation. After Module 1, I discovered that when I was too tired to visualise but I could still read, reading the course books gave a similar energetic experience as visualising the practices.

When writing the portfolios for Module 2 practices I discovered that writing about yoga practices also had an energetic effect. Each time I sat to write about a yoga practice it was like doing the practice all over again and I could describe the effects on my body, the problems I had with it and the alignment points to be aware of; it was like being back in module.

Now I had four ways of doing yoga: visualising, physical practice, reading and writing.

My stamina was improving, as was my balance and my digestion. My eyes were still problematic but at least they were stable.

At the same time, my chakra assignment had been returned, asking me to resubmit – apparently I hadn't sufficiently covered some key points. I disagreed and once again found my pride. I had written my chakra assignment as a personal then societal journey through the chakras, moving from the symptoms of imbalance to the signs of balance.

Initially I thought I would just do the minimal, a table of facts, and resubmit but as soon as I started to research again I realised I couldn't just do the minimal. Fuelled by the chakra dharanam experiences I was having every night, I decided to keep a scrapbook and write about them in synchronicity with my internal learning.

In yogic knowledge, chakras are wheels of energy at key 'intersections' of the body. The seven major chakras are situated along the spinal cord and control the energy flow through specific systems of organs and tissues. Each chakra is also associated with a set of emotional/psychological aspects so that balance and imbalance are experienced as a range of both physical and emotional characteristics.

When the chakras are in balance we have wellbeing, and when they are out of balance or blocked we have disturbed energy flow, hence unwellness in one form or another.

So now I added reading about chakras to my nightly ritual of putting Nicola to sleep; read to her, read to myself and listen to Chris.

I was getting to know my energy system from the inside. It was absolutely fascinating to get to know my body and emotions from the inside in this way. I began to feel the chakras in my body and recognised the concept of energy flow from my continued work with visualisation.

I began to feel like I was really getting to know myself.

EBR2 begins with a series of movements and breathing patterns designed to awaken our creativity, open our heart and warm up our spine. The postures in the second half are mainly concerned with moving energy trapped in the lower chakras; we pump energy up from the base and it moves through a clear spine and into an open heart, to be transformed, ending in Crocodile (**Crocodile** p.173) so we can release what needs to be released and ground the energy we have moved.

It is truly awesome.

In terms of Dru knowledge, this means we are unblocking energy related to security and emotional turbulence; the seat of addictions and attachments. Well, no shortage of that required here. It is such a lovely sequence to practice in its fullness, with a perfect balance of softness and physicality.

It stretches the whole body in every direction and for me it was so lovely even to think about stretching my body in this way, and the times I could manage it physically were bliss.

In terms of walking holy grails, mine came sometime in October. A friend came to take me to a cafe in town. This woman had been a stalwart in my life since 2003 and so it was entirely appropriate that she should be a part of this most significant moment in my life.

Instead of going in the chair, I made the bold move of asking her to put my walker in the back of her car, "Maybe I might walk home, today". If I felt ok after our beverage, I would walk; if I felt like crap, I walk not – simple! She was less than convinced but humoured me.

I used the walker to get from the car to the cafe (so far, so good), and then recovered during chai and cake (at least it was gluten-free). Then I got up to walk home.

"Are you sure you'll be OK?"

"No, I'm not sure but I'm going anyway."

It was the sweetest walk of my life. (and probably the longest). I stopped every few metres to realign my energy as I had done on previous walks but this time I noticed something I had not before. As I realigned the energy through my legs, I noticed a ripple effect through my entire system. It was quite literally like the air around me rippled and shimmered slightly; my breath slowed and deepened, my emotions calmed and my mind cleared.

I felt connected through the layers of my being in a way I had never experienced before, outside of meditation or those moments of peace that occur at extraordinary moments in life. It was amazing to me to be present at the moment of the ripple and to have the awareness of having created the ripple by my own action. This time it wasn't an accident, I could actually 'do' this.

Again that feeling of unstoppableness (after I recovered from the fatigue – there was a cost). I want more! Unfortunately, this also brought with it an anxiety and grasping to do more and go further. My peace and presence was being disturbed by the future again.

It was at this point I started to talk to Trish and Andrew. They were both amazed that I was walking and very enthusiastic so I started giving them regular email updates, something I continue to this day.

Each time I achieved a milestone, walked further and further down the road toward town and back, I would write an email to shout to the world.

Andrew and I made an arrangement for a phone interview about his journey through Chronic Fatigue Syndrome (CFS). The plan was for me to write an article about his use of yoga to manage CFS. The article has never been written but during the interview he said something that changed the way I looked at and worked with walking.

During his recovery he learned to *walk to the beat of his heart.* As soon as he said it I knew it was important, and after the conversation I sat thinking for some time what that might mean for me. "Walking to the beat of my heart?"

What it meant for me at the time was to match the pace of my steps to my own body's rhythm; to tune into my body's rhythm and work in synchronicity with it instead of struggling against it – to go at my own pace.

At first I only applied the teaching to walking but it was such a powerful practice I expanded the application to writing and preparing food and other mundane tasks.

Since then I have learned to apply this invaluable teaching to every aspect of my life. In fact I am relearning it as I write now.

Why was it so important?

It was important for me because I like speed, someone else's speed. Not fast cars or other high adrenalin activities but thinking quickly, learning quickly, walking quickly etc. I grew up as the youngest and smallest of a large family and always felt like I was the slowest, weakest runt of the litter. My own rhythm was never enough.

In my mind *I* was never enough.

Yet the truth of my situation at this time was that I couldn't do more, I couldn't even do what I was trying to do, and the discrepancy was causing so much struggle and angst.

This struggle had crept into walking without me even realising. What had started as a joyful experiment was becoming another 'not enough' struggle. This was such a crucial step in my recovery because it drew my attention to my condition in any given moment and required (still does) a level of acceptance of my condition that broached no argument.

The power of becoming so aware of my body, of accepting and working with what I had/have, is astonishing.

The next day I went walking with my walker again but instead of fighting to take bigger steps and walk further, I relaxed, let go of time and listened to my body. I took tiny steps, sometimes shuffling, often stopping but I got all the way into town and all the way home – the furthest distance I had walked – and the only difference was walking to the beat of my heart.

The joy was overwhelming, because I had walked, but also because I had allowed myself to be me. This was a glimpse of what was possible with acceptance, whatever 'I am' means. The sense of achievement is the same as achieving any other goal.

Next was carrots.

As I said earlier, my hands had worsened and doing any meal preparation was really difficult. I had a carer a couple of times a week to help with meal preparation but the rest of the week was somewhat challenging. I would drop, curse, cut myself, spill, curse and splash, and generally create mayhem. We always ate but the general process was entertaining, to say the least.

After walking to the beat of my heart I discovered I could also slice to the beat of my heart. I know it sounds weird but I'll explain by example. My normal, pre-MS style of slicing vegetables was fast and fine; using the left hand to stabilise the vegetable with fingers tucked in and the right hand holding a very sharp knife, slicing as finely as possible.

All good when things are good but as my hands deteriorated this became more and more farcical. You'd think after three years with this illness I would have learned that faster isn't always better, but no, I had not.

On this day I was dropping, spilling and cutting myself, and was just about ready to give up when Andrew's voice came into my head, saying, "walking to the beat of my heart". So I stopped and breathed; and on the out-breath I imagined my river of gold flowing through my arms and visualised slicing carrots, slowly… and began again.

This time I was very conscious, very present, slicing the carrots, slowly. The whole carrot was sliced before I knew it, without incident and without cursing.

Again.

I peeled another one and did the same thing.

Again it worked so I did it again … and again (we ate a lot of carrots that night). There was such stillness in the air.

Then I began stirring and other preparations with the same stillness and awareness of *doing* at my pace, as it was, with MS.

Dinner was cooked and my mind was so peaceful. There was none of the frustration or struggle I had been experiencing, just the satisfaction of achieving the goal of cooking a meal with ease.

What else?

The more I experimented with this technique, the more ways I found to apply it. Here's another example – completing transactions in shops.

I felt so embarrassed, so often, by my fumbling inability to use money in shops. Sometimes I could feel the impatience of shop attendants and customers, alike, as they waited for me to make my hands work well enough to pay. And of course, the more impatient I became, the worse my hands became.

I have tried so many variations of wallets and

purses, and haven't yet found one that works for me on the days when my hands don't.

So, the next time I was at the supermarket paying for my groceries and found myself fumbling again, the now familiar feeling of panic/embarrassment beginning to rise, and once again Andrew's dulcet tones flowed through my mind.

I stopped, breathed and visualised what I needed to do and then did it: slowly, consciously and with awareness of each movement. The concentration required was enormous but the sense of peace was also enormous, particularly when compared with the struggle I had been experiencing a few moments before.

This is still an issue for me, so if you see me struggling at a supermarket or other retail outlet, please take a deep breath and wait for me to realign my energy into my hands. I may have to concentrate very hard.

After this I started to do more and more things in this way and so I started to be able to do more and more things. The road between my house and the main street became so well known to me and my daughter as I walked, slowly, into town as often as I could. We talked about the changing gardens as we walked and the new flowers as spring blossomed in Braidwood.

Nicola became used to me stopping and stopped asking why, and I graduated from my walker to my Canadian crutches (crutches with callipers around the arms). I still used my chair when I needed to go quickly or felt tired or was going somewhere I might need to stand or wait, or any distance further than my favourite cafe in the main street, but I was walking.

My carers were amazed, my counsellor and physiotherapists were amazed, but the moment it came home to me the most was with Nicola at the local playground.

From the age of 11 months, she had known me in and out of hospital, in wheelchairs or with walking aids, seeing health professionals on a nearly daily basis and being cared for by a range of people who were otherwise strangers.

Trips to the park were in my wheelchair with her on my lap then finding her own way onto and off play equipment, if I was able to get to the park at all. More often she had to wait until someone else could take her.

However, one sunny day in November it was different. We went to the park in my power chair. We arrived at the park and Nicola ran off as usual to play on one of her favourite pieces of equipment. After a short while she asked me to come over to where she was playing.

She had asked me a thousand times before and I had said, "No I'm sorry darling, I can't", but today was different. I got up without sticks and walked over to her.

Nicola looked at me gobsmacked.

"Mum, you're walking, it's a miracle!!!"

Then I realised: in the memory of my four year old this was probably the first time she had seen me walking upright, without sticks.

I cried as I held her close to me at the playground.

Roll on Module 3.

Crocodile

The Crocodile is a beautiful, restorative posture, particularly useful when you are feeling emotionally overwhelmed (trust me, I know about this).

- *Lie on your tummy with your forehead resting on the backs of hands.*
- *Take you feet apart as far apart as is comfortable for you and turn your ankles in towards each other*
- *Let go from your belly, a little bit more with each exhalation.*
- *When you are done, draw your legs back together, bring your bottom back on to your heels and rest in the Child (buttocks resting on your heels, forehead resting on the ground or one fist on top of the other) for a few moments before going to back to your life.*
- *I did not immediately connect with this posture until I laid down on the grass in the sun on our land at Majors Creek. I still remember the sweet smell of the grass and the soil as released of my sense of feeling overwhelmed.*

Module 3

NOVEMBER 2007

My life in the weeks before Module 3 was one of wonder and delight but utterly exhausting. I was still relatively disabled but improving almost daily. I had the feeling that everyone around me was holding their breath, waiting for something to happen, hoping it wouldn't. As I have already said, MS is a bizarre disease and life can change, seemingly in an instant. But for me at this time, it didn't.

Again I procrastinated organising the details and left everything to the last minute, with "should I, shouldn't I" constantly plaguing my thoughts. This has also become a familiar pattern of my life with Dru as I have struggled against the one thing that has consistently improved both my state of mind and my physical wellbeing.

The other question at the forefront of my mind was, "Do I bring the wheelchair or not?"

At that time I was only using it for long distances and public outings where I might need to stand and wait. Distance is so deceptive. A distance that is no trouble for a healthy person, such that you wouldn't even notice it, becomes a marathon or worse for a person with a disability.

It was a difficult decision because pride was competing vehemently with practicality but practicality won; walking once a day and around my house is very different to walking all day, every day. The decisive factor were the trips to the park to yoga in the sun, such a beautiful thing to do and not possible for me without the wheelchair. I took the wheelchair and parked it outside the room and walked into the room.

The reaction of my peers and my teachers over the next four days was a mixture of shock, incredulity and curiosity. It was the most confusing four days of my teacher training.

The first thing was Trish exclaiming at the lovely article that had been written about me and the potential for it being published everywhere. What article?

I had done an interview a few weeks before but I thought it was for a few quotes in an article about the teacher training course and was unaware an article had been written about me.

Then the module started and I started to do yoga with everyone else, and I could feed multiple pairs of eyes on me as I bent and stretched. The balance of my practice had been gradually shifting from visualisation to physical, as my condition improved. I felt such joy in being able to move; and I found that if I visualised and moved at the same time, the movement even became graceful.

I so loved EBR2, visualising and doing, so when we came to practice it in module I just let myself go into the practice. Again, the hours of visualisation had prepared my mind and this time the hours of walking and bits of 'doing' had prepared my body.

So here I was at module moving in my own space and it felt like pure luxury. I closed my eyes and allowed the verbal cues of the teachers to lead my mind and body through the sequence, opening my heart, pumping blocked energy from the base of my spine and then directing it up through my body into my heart, up and out through my crown.

I now teach yoga to a range students with a range of mobility and one of the instructions I give is to "allow your whole body to luxuriate in the movement, even if it is only your finger moving" and another to "move with the excitement of moving for the first time".

These instructions come from this module when I really discovered what it felt like to move for the first time and to luxuriate in my body. I had never experienced a greater pleasure; no food, beverage or sensation could compare with the bliss of finding stillness within movement after months of having to find movement within stillness.

Then the break.

"How did you do it?"

"Are you taking new drugs?"

"You look so strong." Etc, etc, etc.

Every break for the next four days was spent talking about me. I felt so embarrassed, overwhelmed and undeserving of all the attention. I wanted to know about other people's lives and what they had been doing (there were so many interesting people on my course), but they seemed to be more interested in my life. I suddenly felt very conspicuous.

Again there were the same issues for me around personalities and my social skills, and rather than making it easier, my new status seemed to make it more difficult for me. In my mind, the attention made my own inadequacies more obvious.

However, following on from last module I was determined to face my difficulties and extend myself to people I was reacting to – I recommend this as a method of dealing with social situations, as it really does work while making friends with the most unlikely people. There are hidden jewels everywhere.

I was totally unprepared for the attention I was receiving. My ego had craved this kind of attention all my life and was enjoying it. The deeper part of me that felt wrong was totally embarrassed and couldn't understand all the fuss, couldn't accept the praise and felt totally undeserving.

Then there was me that was trying to get my head around what was actually happening in my body. My yoga practice within the module was once again reflecting what was possible. After over 10 years of experiencing dysfunction to some degree in nearly every system of my body, I was functional and flowing, again.

Emotionally, I was confused and a mess!

We weren't having small group mentoring in this module as we had during Module 2. Instead we had one-on-ones with one of the senior tutors. I was booked in with Trish, which was then changed to Andrew which was then changed to the beautiful Monica. I was ambivalent about the mentoring because, while I felt the same dread of talking about my experiences, I was also hanging out to go "BLAH".

So I sat with Monica in the cafe area, drinking chai lattes and really wanting to spill my messy bits but feeling absolutely terrified of doing so. Can you imagine the relief when Monica too wanted to know what I'd been doing? Phew!

And in a way, it was lovely to talk about the previous two months with one of the people who had originally been so influential in me starting the course. Having been the person who had said, "It's OK, you can visualise and you won't be distracted by the physical thing", I could understand why she, more than anyone, would want to know what had happened for me.

As we talked about my practice, and my life that was becoming my practice, my eyes filled with water and the air around us became still. It was like a long exhalation.

Monica said I was giving Reiki with my eyes; another phrase that has changed my perspective on my life. If there is nothing else I can give, I can look at someone with love in my heart and give some healing, even if it is just for the moment.

The practices of Module 3 were perfect. Chandra Namaskara (Chandra meaning moon and Namaskara meaning salute – salute to the moon) I loved instantly. The first time was learning. We practiced several repetitions, slowly and building our understanding of each posture in our bodies and breath. I mixed visualising with physical 'doing'; still not taking notes, I consciously opened my mind on all levels to learn as internally as I could.

The second time of practicing was absolutely transformative. It was the fourth day and we had been yoga-ing and meditating for three and a half days; my emotions and mind were wide open. I felt like I was merging with the sequence, merging with the peaceful serenity of the moon, itself.

Chandra Namaskara is a practice particularly good for soothing and balancing hormonal fluctuations. I have found it particularly useful in managing the mini-exacerbations I have at ovulation and pre-menses. I have heard of a woman who practiced it every day for twelve months to manage menopause; and have recently discovered it is invaluable in managing mood swings not necessarily related to hormone fluctuations at all.

One advantage of not being able to take notes through modules was that when I was learning new techniques, I learned them so deeply that permanent shifts seemed to take place during the learning process.

My body, mind and spirit seemed to undergo their own transformations as I was connecting deeply with the practices to learn them. I felt and still feel that learning in the way I did, have embedded the practices in my mind and body in a way I have never experienced before.

My connection with Chandra Namaskara was so deep as to bring an irregular cycle into synchronicity with the cycle of the moon, almost instantly. My cycle has remained in synchronicity with the moon since, with the exception of a few months of irregular bleeding in 2009.

However, this deep connection on day 4 was also my undoing. It struck at such a deep place I could no longer contain all the conflicting emotions I had been feeling over the last few days.

For the last two and a half months I had been so focussed on my practice, both yoga and life, I had forgotten to notice I was achieving the 'impossible'. Yet in the last four days, my peers, teachers and practice were reflecting exactly that. I wanted to tell them that they could do what I had done – it was nothing special – but I didn't get the opportunity. I didn't feel like I had done anything special, I felt like I was just doing what I had been told (for once).

I found a quiet place with a good friend (who had herself defeated the odds by surviving 'terminal' breast cancer) and the dam burst; days, weeks and months of emotion overflowed. I sobbed and sobbed until I was done. There were no words and still aren't.

In less than six months my yoga and meditation practice had taken me from wheelchair dependent to barely using my sticks, let alone my wheelchair. I stood straight and could make it through most days without needing a disco nap. I could eat a meal without excruciating pain afterwards and I could speak and, most importantly to me, could think again.

So, why did I still feel like a fraud?

The Testimonial

DECEMBER 2007

The hangover from Module 3 was in direct proportion to the turbulence of the module itself. I arrived home feeling like I was only half done. I wanted to return to the module and complete it but it had all been packed up and was just an empty function room now. The oasis of the module was now just a mirage in my memory.

It's funny but you'd think with all emotional turbulence and physical aches and pains that come with yoga modules, we would be desperate to get home and return to some stability and comfort. Yet most of us found it difficult to leave and looked forward to the next time we would be seeing each other. I have often wondered why.

Now I wonder if the positive, warm and supportive environment that is so carefully created by the tutors and support staff enabled us to forebear the discomforts and distress we experience, and even anticipate it with joy. Then I wonder if we could apply this to the rest of life and what a difference it might make.

For me this time there was one big question. How do I integrate all that had happened and been realised, into a life with three children, a husband and maths students?

The answer was just to do it: love my children, draw them close and be with them; teach my maths students and talk to my husband. We had again grown distant. He spent most weekends on our land, building, and I was still in too much emotional pain to go out there much, and during the week I went to bed with Nicola and chakra dharanam straight after dinner.

A week or so after the module I opened my inbox to find the testimonial that had been written about my story. At first I couldn't bring myself to read it. "What if I liked it?" "What if I didn't like it?" "What if …" I'm not sure which outcome I was more afraid of or even why it was an issue but it was an issue; it's hard to admit to such a senseless waste of energy based in pride and ego.

It sat in my inbox for a couple of days until I could bear to click open. Even when I did begin reading, I had to stop several times to let the welling emotions subside. Why? I still don't know. It was just such an overwhelming feeling reading about me, written by someone else. It was real but it seemed so unreal.

When the emotions finally subsided I found two thoughts remained; the testimonial was well written and it wasn't me. Before I had a chance to install a control, another thought embedded itself, "I will have to write it myself."

Oh my god, what have I just agreed to? I hadn't said it aloud, I could choose not to do it but I knew in that simple mind statement I had committed myself to a course of action I am still following today; that ultimately resulted in this book.

That seemingly small decision to write my own testimonial, made partly out of reaction, part arrogance, part attachment and part sattva (sattva is a Sanskrit word meaning pure intention) changed my life almost as much as the one to do the teacher training course.

How the **** do I write about my journey when I don't even know what I did? What do I include? What do I leave out? So began the angst that seemed to last for weeks (it must have only been 1-2 weeks but it seemed like forever). I made several beginnings in several different notebooks, at different times; each one with an essence of truth but seeming false to me and not quite right. When I finally sat down to write I discarded them all in the hope that all the perceived pretention was also being discarded.

As I sat at my keyboard I meditated on the highest outcome, the highest good for all. This has become a ritual for me since when writing anything about yoga, and later, anything contentious. Of course, I have forgotten at times of extreme emotion but whenever I remembered, the outcome was always conciliatory when it could have been conflict or a more eloquent piece of writing than I thought I could produce.

However, even with the meditation, writing my testimony was like pulling teeth. The actual writing took two days over a weekend as I tried to retain the truth of the previous attempts and expand on what I thought was important, in a way that didn't make me wince.

Finally it was done and I sent it to a friend I knew would be both honest and accurate. The wait was agonising but finally she called with her revisions. We sat on the phone for an hour, her at her computer and me at mine, and tweaked my writing until we were both happy. Phew, I wasn't a wanker, at least in her eyes.

The testimony was 2,199 words, far too long for what Dru wanted, but I couldn't edit any more. Now to send it on; more angst and more procrastination. I had an underlying sense that sending this would have a dramatic effect on my life. Of course, I had no real concept what the effect might be; only that it would bring about change. The little saboteur in my head was again deriding me for being pretentious, "it was nothing, and no-one will be interested".

Finally, I sat in silence in front of my computer and asked the question. "Send or not send?" "Send!" the answer came with such strong compulsion, I immediately pressed 'send'; one to Andrew, one to Trish and one to the person who had written the original testimonial (with an apology).

It was done.

"Oh my God, what have I done?"

The Camel Waits While the Dancer Salutes the Moon

DECEMBER 2007 CONTINUED

A few weeks before the module, I had started doing a posture we hadn't yet learned. I must have learned it in a previous yoga class or seen someone doing it, although I couldn't remember where, it just seemed to come out of me somehow. When I described it to Trish she said it is 'the Dancer', a master asana, and one of its benefits is to remove emotional blocks.

"Yep, I can do with some of that."

I loved doing it (and still do) and did it whenever I could. Sometimes I couldn't hold it for very long, sometimes I needed to hold on to something and sometimes I had to visualise, but regardless of how much I needed to modify the posture, it always felt amazing.

It was with the Dancer I really learnt the value of

relaxing in the posture and letting the prana hold me. I would get into whatever version of the posture I could (this even works with visualising, or especially with visualising) and relax my body and relax my mind, and go inside into the stillness.

So how happy was I to see it in the course book for module 3?

The Dancer focuses awareness on the lower abdomen and sacrum. We learnt the posture outside under the trees, visualising water running through our lower abdomen/sacrum area. In Dru yoga this area relates to emotional turbulence and attachments, so visualising water running through this area is cleansing, particularly if practiced after a heart opening exercise. The emotion released from the sacrum moves up into the heart, is transformed and released.

How wonderful to be asked to practice a posture my body wanted to do anyway.

In all Dru practices there is a moment where stillness is found within movement, the still point around which the whole asana or sequence revolves; when motion becomes meditation. For me at this point of my journey, the Dancer was a still point in itself and the still point within Dancer was the centre around which my whole life seemed to revolve; a key to eternity.

Then on Christmas Eve I went on a picnic with my family, by a beautiful river which winds through a nearby national park.

First we *walked* down to the river, no chair or walker or sticks, just my children, my mum, Matthew and me. Then we stopped at a bend in the river; water rushing past, little eddies of water around a rock shelf jutting out into the river just at the tip of the elbow.

I stood on the edge of the rock feeling the euphoria of unaided verticalness. I had always loved rock edges and never thought I would stand on one again but here I was standing safely watching the river. I found myself thinking the Dancer, feeling the energy beginning to move through my body. My breathing changed, the air around me changed and the now familiar feeling of peace began to permeate my awareness.

"Why not do it?"

"OK"

And I did (*The Dancer* p.195). It is so easy to change my state of mind. Nothing in my external environment had changed but in a few minutes my whole perspective on my life in this moment had shifted. This was happening more and more in my life and it never ceased to amaze me.

The rest of the day passed in a surreal haze of serenity, so unusual for Christmas Eve. We returned to the picnic site and finished our picnic. I felt connected even to the ants carrying the crumbs of our Christmas cake back to their nest. I felt joy in every moment, no matter how mundane.

Just before Christmas, a couple of friends had loaned me two books that were to become important in my healing; the *Power of Now* by Eckhart Tolle and *the Journey* by Brandon Bays. They were revelatory for two very different reasons. Tolle talked theory about the importance of presence and the irrelevance of past and future; how we accumulate a pain body through our lives by not being present and the importance of releasing pain as we go.

Many times while reading through the pages of Tolle's writing I found myself saying, "Yes, that's me" or "I wonder if I can do that".

Bays, on the other hand, tells her own story of working through successive major life crises, including an abdominal growth, using alternative methods such as diet and body work, all the while refining a process of dealing with past trauma. The process works on resolving buried trauma in order to heal the physical/psychological/behavioural dysfunction resulting from the trauma.

Through the book, Bays not only uses her own history as an example but cites several cases where significant physical or psychological dysfunction have been healed, using this process. She was inspired by people who had healed themselves before her and was offering her own story in the same way.

I knew the mind had incredible power to heal, both from my earlier experience with asthma and my current experiences with MS, but here were two different perspectives saying the same thing – you can have a significant role in healing yourself.

A coincidence, maybe … or maybe not.

Regardless, Tolle escaped the psychological torture of depression and Bays resolved an abdominal tumour so it must be possible for me to transform my own madness.

I was still reading the Gita and hearing her message of non-attachment and the associated freedom (it is only now I am realising just how difficult true non-attachment really is) and the combination inspired me to see what I could do; to see what I could release.

So still in a meditative state from the picnic, I decided Christmas Eve was the time. I had gone to sleep late without my usual ritual with Nicola, due to last minute present wrapping (a Christmas ritual with my husband) and general Christmas jolliness.

My mind was busy as I tossed and turned between Matthew and Nicola so I did what had almost become automatic – I did yoga in my mind. Instantly I became calmer and my busy mind settled. I was able to give myself a deep relaxation but still felt wide awake.

It occurred to me to try the Journey myself. This was probably not recommended but my natural arrogance thought, "Why not".

I was already in a state of relaxation and months of working with my mind, combined with some deep yogic breath, enabled me to reach a point where I was able to step into the boat of my unconscious.

I asked the boat to take me to the part of my body in most need of healing.

The first place we went was my heart where I felt quite sharp pain. The issue, from my childhood, was seemingly trivial but using techniques from both my yoga training and the Journey the issue was soon resolved and off we went to the next destination.

This was the beginning of what seemed like hours

of cruising through my body to sites of stored unresolved issues collected along my life. It was incredibly painful at times, to the point of panic but I continued using a combination of breath techniques we had learned in module 3 (*Module 3 Breath Techniques* p.196) and an affirmation.

On my tour through my body on Christmas Eve I breathed around the square and used the affirmation "I am love now" to divide the breath into fractions and keep all the phases even.

What amazes me about that night was the triviality of the issues and the pain they were causing; it really is the little things that count. It was bizarre.

To put this in context, I had been plagued through my life by revisiting painful, humiliating and disempowering moments, in dreams, nightmares and daydreams. I had no idea they were being stored throughout my body (although, I wonder if they are actually stored in the corresponding parts of our brain and the body is where they are expressed).

Compared to what I had experienced over the last couple of years, these issues seemed insignificant. Yet it wasn't the big things in my life that appeared that Christmas Eve, it was the little slights to my ego, over and over again, at all different ages, in all different circumstances. How easily I was offended, how reactive I was and now I was finding out exactly how much pain they were causing.

I don't think I slept much that night but I woke on Christmas day lighter than I remembered feeling, almost dizzy with the lightness of being. I remember wondering if those stories would return to plague me again and decided to just enjoy this moment without them. However, in the time hence, not one of these stories has returned, in dream or daydream, and many of the behaviours they generated are falling away.

I was gobsmacked when I realised in such a graphic way how much baggage I had been carrying and how heavy it made me feel. I vowed to begin a process of letting go as I go along. I don't always succeed and I continue to find stories that were not released that night or since but the intention is strong and I definitely feel lighter as I go on.

As I reflect on this experience, Christmas Eve 2007 was a before and after moment where life is significantly different after.

And this brings me to the camel. When we learnt the camel posture in module, I couldn't do the full posture; my thighs weren't strong enough to hold me up for any length of time, my shoulders were too tight, and the joints of my toes too tight and sore to curl under for the preliminary stage.

Even still, I strained my shoulder trying to push myself into it (yes, I know – naughty) because I knew there was something about the camel I wanted. It looked like the whole chest opened and I really wanted to experience that kind of openness. Eventually I surrendered and visualised.

Wow, how beautiful. I was right, there was something in the Camel I wanted and it was this extraordinary opening of the chest. I sat in the posture in my mind and felt warmth moving up from the base of my spine and light streaming out of my heart.

It was enough to draw me on. When I got home I visualised the front of my body opening, my shoulders loosening and my quads strengthening, as well as a lot of physical stretches for my shoulders. Day after day I worked with my mind, imagining muscle fibres lengthening and invisible hands lifting my ribcage higher and holding me in the posture.

When I visualised the posture, my sternum was pointing straight up; of course, in physical reality my sternum was nowhere near pointing up but my mind was capable of perfection.

The lungs are sometimes referred to as a storehouse of grief and sadness, so when we open our chest like we do in the camel, we make it possible to release some of those stored feelings of grief and sadness. For me it was also a feeling of being exposed and I wanted to feel that freedom so I could walk with an open heart.

Finally, one day soon after Christmas, a thought came into my head to try the camel again. I hadn't attempted it physically since the module because I had hurt my shoulder so much. I wanted to wait until I could do it without pain.

I spent some time warming up my body and doing the specific body preps for the posture. "OK, now or never." (*Camel* p.197)

I felt so excited, so emotional and teary. I didn't hold the posture for very long and came down into the posture of the Child, but for the moments I was in it, I was invincible. My body had let go enough over Christmas to enable me to go into the full camel. What a gift!

Did the hours of visualising before Christmas loosen the niggley things to be released on Christmas Eve or did the release of the niggley things on Christmas Eve loosen the joints, generating greater flexibility and enabling me to move into the Camel?

Probably both: the yoga loosened the hold so the stuff could be released and the release created more space in the muscles and joints, generating greater flexibility and strength.

Writing now it is hard to imagine the tortured girl who constantly lived in the wounds of her past.

She seems like someone else I knew once.

The Dancer

- *I stood in Tadasana and breathed*
- *Engaged core stability and took my weight on my left leg, anchoring the left foot into the rock shelf*
- *Raised my right knee and slid the right hand down my right thigh and around to my right ankle.*
- *Held my ankle behind my ankle, got my balance, breathe, rose up out of the hips, lengthened through my spine out of the crown. Raised the left hand and formed the njaan mudra.*
- *The peace began to descend as my awareness went inwards and sank to the space between*

---

my lower abdominal wall and my sacrum
- *Began to pivot from the hips*
- *Extended the left hand out in front while extending the right leg behind*
- *Now, lengthened through the whole body and relaxed.*
- *Surrender, stillness, rest.*
- *At this point my lower abdomen seemed to open and I felt like I was merging with the river as it passed through this centre, cleansing as it flowed.*
- *My mind felt so much clearer and deeply calm, time seemed to stop.*
- *I came out of the posture in the reverse order and moved into the other side.*
- *The same merging feeling and the tranquillity deepened.*

Module 3 Breath Techniques

Samra vritti *is a breathing technique that involves breathing in for a count (e.g. four), holding for the same count, breathing out for the same count and holding for the same count. Another term for samra vritti is 'square breathing'. Square breathing alters the consciousness slightly while bringing extraordinary clarity and calm.*

*   **Viloma breath** is also called 'fractional breathing' because it breaks the in and out-*

breath into even fractions. It measures the breath and hence brings measure and control to the mind.

Caution: Introducing new breathing patterns should always be done gradually with caution and if any discomfort such as dizziness or light-headedness is felt, one should return immediately to a normal breathing pattern.

Camel

- I came into standing kneeling with the front of my feet flat on the floor.
- Raised my right arm in an arc in front of me, continuing the arc behind until my hand rested on my right heel.
- Raised my left arm in the same way until my left hand was also resting on my heel
- The same invisible hands underneath my ribcage lifted my spine up out of my hips, pushing my hips slightly forward and taking the weight off my thighs
- Surrender and relax
- And then the light came.

I felt so excited, so emotional and teary. I didn't hold the posture for very long and came down into the posture of the child but for the moments I was in it, I was invincible. My body had let go enough over Christmas to enable me go into the full camel. What a gift!

Giving Energy

NEW YEAR'S EVE 2007

It was around this time I started to become aware the incident with my friends' neck was not isolated. I had no idea what I was doing (still don't really) and the only evidence I had that I was in fact doing anything at all was the difference in how I felt and what the people involved said was happening for them. Oh, and that there was some improvement in their condition.

One of my fondest memories from childhood was sitting behind my sister on Thursday nights after she came home from work, brushing her hair and massaging her shoulders while she handed around the Rocky Road she had bought from the Darrell Lea shop she passed on the way home. I didn't even like Rocky Road but I loved to massage my sister's shoulders (I still love massaging her shoulders every time I stay with her).

I have always loved tactile contact with people and

this became a tradition. I did a massage course with mum at her university a couple of years later because I thought I wanted to be a physiotherapist and continued massaging whenever I could.

People groan when I massage but everyone groans when they get massages and I didn't think I was any better than anyone else; I just loved doing it, and when my children came along they loved it too.

I wasn't entirely convinced by the concept of energy healing and even with the understanding of energy in the body I now have; I still think the practitioner has to be very clear to be effective in moving energy just by laying on hands. So here I was noticing that people were feeling something when I put my hands on them (other than my hands – ha–ha). They described a range of sensations, including unusual warmth, and pins and needles etc, but most commonly felt soothed and calmed.

My own feet often ached with stiffness and when I placed my hands over them, they were also soothed and softened. It often made the difference between walking and not walking. I found I could do this with any part of my body (any part I could reach – another good reason for doing yoga).

So when my husband came home from the Creek the day before New Year's Eve with spasms in his back, in agonising pain, I thought, "why not". He lay down and I placed my hands on his back and breathed in a pattern that occurred to me on the spot.

This certainly wasn't an intellectual exercise.

I breathed in through the crown, into my heart; out of my heart, down through my right hand; into my left hand up into my heart; down into the earth; up into my heart, out through my right hand; into my left up into my heart and out through the crown. Repeatedly… for an hour.

He wasn't cured but he was soothed and I felt remarkably peaceful. That night he tossed and turned and finally woke up unable to get back to sleep so I did it again. This time he was soothed into a calm sleep. Every time the pain became too much for him to bear, I would place my hands on his back, he would go to sleep and I would also feel transformed.

We had planned a trip down to the coast for New Year's Eve and when he woke in the morning still in pain we didn't think we would make it, but after another session of my hands, he decided to go. We loaded up the car and drove down the mountain.

Of course that was the other small issue – Matthew couldn't drive due to the back pain and I hadn't driven for months due to MS. Blind arrogance on my part again as I assured everyone I would be fine. I meditated before we left and climbed into the driver's seat with an open mind (and my fingers crossed).

A break at Bateman's Bay and some yoga in my mind, and anti inflammatory tablets for Matthew, and we were off again. The concentration demanded to keep my body from going off line was remarkable.

We stopped two more times to give both Matthew and myself a break but it was amazing the peace I felt.

I needed to meditate while I was driving and of course this gave me that same sense of peace that yoga and meditation always did. The best way to describe this process is keeping my mind, hence body, completely relaxed and open, yet alert.

So when we arrived at my friend's house at some time in the afternoon, after being on the road most of the day, I felt invincible again; completely exhausted but invincible.

What a way to start the New Year.

I continued to work on Matthew's back over the following days and he gradually recovered. He may have recovered anyway but it was lovely to give him some comfort in the meantime. And for me it was lovely to discover two new paths to freedom; meditating in order to drive and giving.

Reaching Out for the Fruit at the End of the Branch

JANUARY 2008

So begins 2008 with a camping holiday to the coast and doings of the impossible, crossing boundaries of physical activity previously thought uncrossable.

I walked along a bush track to the lagoon and back, not just once but several times during our week of camping. The track is 500m each way, a 1km round trip. This may not sound much if you are able bodied but for me who only recently was able to walk from the front door to the back and into the backyard without sticks, it was a miracle.

After the first trip I arrived back at the campsite and crashed on to the floor of our kitchen tent, sleeping for two hours, but it didn't matter because I had done the undoable. Seven months before I didn't think I would ever walk any distance again.

After this, I took any opportunity to walk to the lagoon, sometimes carrying Nicola for short distances, sometimes resting in the shade but always with the alertness of someone living the impossible. It was like having the heightened vision and hearing of someone who has just cheated death to be amongst the living again but with a new awareness of what that actually means.

Then I thought I would do something completely ridiculous and ride a bike. The loss of my balance was something I had mourned (and still do sometimes) because I had appreciated having good balance (no, really I had hubris around having good balance). So I mounted the bike with Grace next to me, Matthew watching me from behind and Nicola complaining because I couldn't take her with me.

Then I rode to the toilet block! It was a bit wobbly and to anyone watching I probably looked like a silly middle-aged woman trying and not succeeding to be young again, but for me it was the Olympics and I was crossing the line first. Then I rode back. Was it just me or did I notice a tear in Matthew's eyes? There were plenty in mine and one or two in Grace's too.

I maintained my yoga practice getting up in the morning and going to the beach to meditate and do yoga. Two days in a row I saw dolphins playing in the waves and swimming in the sea further out. Then at night I went again to salute the rising moon with Chandra Namaskara.

Walking to the beach was a practice in itself because I frequently had to stop and move energy around my body before I could move on; stopping halfway up the stairs to rest leaden legs, and halfway down for fear of falling the rest of the way.

Having decided to share more intimately my growing practice with Matthew, one night I invited him to join me on the beach. He had not seen me practice physically very much and only in the context of our daily life (a posture while cooking dinner or on the lounge room floor while watching television), so it had never had the same intensity as yoga in module or my private practice. I felt very, very nervous, like I was exposing an intimate part of myself, but I wanted him to know me.

We had fallen in to the trap of many married couples, particularly those who have suffered trauma: we stopped communicating. After we returned from Britain we seemed to adopt a policy of avoiding any topic of conversation that might lead to the emotional aspects of MS, or, in fact, any other emotional aspects of anything.

MS (and the other events of the previous few years) hung between us like an invisible veil and I had begun to feel like I was on my own with the management of this illness.

I like to think I tried to broach the subject(s) but now I wonder how much I tried and if I gave up too quickly. Regardless, give up I did. We fell into the habit of divided lives under the same roof. He went to 'Creek' most weekends and worked during the week, while I continued on with my tasks.

In the period since Module 3 I had realised I had to be the partner I wanted and vowed to share this world that was opening up for me. So on the beach that night I showed him who I was becoming. I wanted to bridge some of the yawning chasm that had grown between us but now I wonder if I made it bigger.

He sat some distance away on the beach and watched as once again I saluted the glorious waxing moon as it rose over the ocean. I forgot Matthew was watching and allowed all my gratitude to pour into the sequence.

At one point, in a twist looking up at my right hand, I saw a flock of birds flying across the sky in the perfect shape of a chevron; such a blessing. I felt a deep connection with Chandra, as the moon is called in Sanskrit, and the deep serenity accompanied by her subterranean power.

When I finished, Matthew came to sit with me and was very quiet. My first thought was that old habitual pattern of thinking anyone else's silence indicated I had done something wrong. I couldn't have been more wrong; he was awestruck by the power of the sequence. He said I 'glowed', and I think he started to get the connection between my practice and me – it wasn't something I *did* but something I *was*.

As we walked back to the campsite, something was different between us; he understood something about me he hadn't before and I felt more freedom to express the ooby-gooby bits of myself.

We both felt a heightened awareness and connection to the natural world around us. I felt like I could almost hear the water moving within the trees (who'd have thunk I would have been so ooby-gooby) and couldn't have deliberately caused harm to another being.

The rest of the holiday was marked by moments of connection with each of my three children. Reading and playing with Nicola, listening to Gabriel talk about his girlfriend and Grace with the rising of the moon telling me she wanted to go to Canberra for years 9-12, pre-empting our eventual move to the 'big smoke'.

Her explanation was so well reasoned, while recognising she needed to complete some things in Braidwood. I couldn't help but feel respect for this twelve-year-old girl who was making such a mature request with such forward planning. Immediately I began to think about ways we could achieve it for her.

By the end of our week at the beach I began to contemplate being strong and capable again. It was thrilling and exciting and tantalisingly close. The perfectly ripe piece of fruit at the end of the branch, too far to reach but maybe if I stretched just a little bit further I might be able to pick it and eat it.

The Journey

JANUARY 2008

Soon after we returned, from our holiday, I was lucky enough to meet someone who was just finishing her practitioners training in the Journey. All that was needed was case studies, and curious to do the real thing, I offered to be one of these. We sat and talked while we ate and I clarified the question I wanted answered.

Finally we began our journey into the deeper recesses of my mind. My question was around feeling unacknowledged in a recent situation. In my waking mind it was impossible to get any perspective on the situation because I had so many loud conflicting emotions. I didn't want to need other people's approval so I fought and resented the intrusion, and I couldn't get into a quiet enough space on my own to hear the underlying truth.

Feeling unappreciated and unacknowledged has been a lifelong issue for me and this was just one example of the thought habit. It was to be another two years before I was able to get to the bottom of the need for external acknowledgement, but this was the first step to unravelling this particular tangle. It also gave me a stronger sense of the power of going below the chaos of our everyday monkey mind – the chattering noise of our everyday thoughts.

The Four Threads of My Tapestry

JANUARY – MARCH 2008

Over the few years since my time in Britain, I had come to look at my life as a tapestry, with many threads weaving in and out to make the whole picture of my life. When I see this in my mind's eye it is a huge wall hanging telling a rich story of love, lightness and darkness, of many different colours and shades; like the Bayeux Tapestries of France. And just like in a tapestry, there is no good and bad, there is only 'what is'.

At this time there were four main threads in my life, interweaving to create the one scene: the books I was reading to open my mind and heart to what was possible; my practice, both yoga and nascent meditation; my family, including my children and my relationship with my husband, as well as my mother at this time; and my students.

MS wove its way through all of these threads but increasingly as a background theme rather than the main colour it had been. I was still being supported by carers because my condition was still highly variable (showering could still bring me undone) and everyone was waiting for the relapse.

The care funding program we had applied for when I first had my relapse in 2006 had been approved, in part, over the Christmas period but I could no longer in all integrity accept it because my condition no longer justified full-time care.

It was bizarre. My family and I desperately needed consistent 7-day assistance over the first 18 months after my relapse and the framework for providing the funding for this kind of care was there but the bureaucracy involved in accessing the funding was such that my application took over 18 months to manifest into an offer.

Not to mention that the offer finally made wasn't for the program of self-management for which we originally applied; and this was due to the decision of a reviewing person halfway through the application process, who didn't listen to my needs, believing she knew better – she didn't, neither did she inform me of her decision.

The original program involved managing the funding and employing the carers myself, through an agency based in Sydney. This meant I would be able to interview and negotiate directly with the carers, myself – a very personalised and empowering solution to the challenge of providing care for the intimate needs of the chronically disabled.

I am deeply grateful for the care I received because without it we would have been even more desperate. However, needing the sort of intimate care I did is incredibly disempowering and I am sure you can all imagine having the right to negotiate how that care is delivered, when and by who, would introduce some dignity into the concept of needing someone else to wipe your bum, literally and metaphorically.

This is not a new concept, someone had not only conceived it but set up the framework. The problem was accessing it and convincing well-meaning public servants that it was a good idea.

How many places can you put a cheese grater?

Does a cheese grater go in the saucepans cupboard because it's metal or does it go with the strainers and sieves and miscellaneous kitchen equipment because it's miscellaneous? It could go with the bowls (not sure why) or it could go in the plastics (not sure why, either, perhaps because many things we can't place go in the plastics cupboard).

Then of course, once we have decided on the cupboard, which shelf?

These and many other similar dilemmas are the reasons why it would often take us many minutes and rummaging through every cupboard and shelf (and the drawers) to find the simplest of things, particularly the cheese grater. With a different carer every day and some days, two different carers on the same day, finding things in our cupboards was a constant puzzle.

"Why would you put that there?"

If we said this in exasperated tones, once a day, we said it twenty times. And for some reason the cheese grater was the thing most commonly 'lost'. The myriad of possibilities was astounding, not only between people but sometimes the same people. Kitchen items would go missing for weeks only to turn up while hunting for something else in the most seemingly unlikely place.

Interestingly, it was my family who had the most difficulty with the ever changing nature of our kitchen cupboards. Perhaps I was a little more used to it, having lived with people who never put the same thing in the same place, twice – them! At one stage Matthew even threatened labelling the shelves. I laughed knowing it would make no difference to the carers or to my family.

For me, having so many carers in my house was a little like getting a peek into the psychology of others. Seeing the variety of ways people hang clothes on the line, wash up or organise kitchen cupboards. There were also many different ways in which people showered and dressed me; from quick and business-like to soft and nurturing.

Some people went through the house like lightning, doing as much as possible, and others took a long time on particular tasks. Some liked to talk, others were more silent. It was fascinating to watch how many different ways there were to do seemingly simple tasks and how ingrained these ways become.

It was also fascinating to see how attached we are to our own way of doing things and how disempowering it is to have someone else come into your house and do your domestics, their way. It feels like your life is being taken over. I had no idea I was this attached.

Clothes on the line and how they were folded were constant sources of angst for me. One would think being in a wheelchair would have put things into perspective but somehow the creases in my clothes was still of great importance. And do you think I could ask for it to be done my way? I felt trivial and small for even being concerned. It is difficult enough to accept the help, let alone have the power to guide the process. So I angsted.

Then one day a carer who had become a friend and said she had changed her own ways as a result of a client asking her to do something differently, and had not been offended at all.

It was a subtle way of telling me I could tell my carers what I wanted without offending and I might even be of help.

It worked and I began to regain a sense of control in my house. I began to ask for what I wanted, and as I did so it became less important – it was the idea of self-determination not the actual tasks.

And perhaps it might be useful for people to understand that while someone is disabled, they are still in their own home and that it might be nice to ask how they like their washing put out.

I have never thought of myself as attached to doing my own housework or having territorial aspects to my domestic role but I was and I did. What I found was having a little self-determination allowed me to let go of 'my way' and embrace the myriad of 'other ways'.

Even so, when I began to do my own domestic tasks again, it was such a joy. I remember feeling overjoyed to iron, because I could. I would iron our clothes with great satisfaction and have the ironing board set up for days. Fortunately this hasn't lasted. Piles of neatly folded washing made me supremely happy (embarrassingly, this has stuck). Washing up became fun (when I could do it again without breaking stuff), and putting away dishes is still slightly comical. Vacuuming is still a trial and I look forward to the day when this simple task also fills me with joy, but sweeping is deeply satisfying. And I love being able to serve people in my own house because I can.

And it matters less how things are done or where they are put; I am increasingly grateful they are done somehow and put somewhere.

So, how many places can you put a cheese grater?

As many places as there are cupboards and shelves within cupboards in the kitchen.

And where does the cheese grater go in my kitchen, now? Wherever it fits!

Family

Anyway, the consistent theme of my tapestry was my family; no matter what else happens in my life, I always have my family. However, at this time, my family were providing their own challenges.

First, my youngest was off to school. Absolute heartache. We had been so close through the ordeal of MS (and everything else) but I needed to send her into the world. Our circumstances since her birth had been such that we had been socially isolated, and while her relating to adults was exceptional due to the cast of thousands involved in my care, she needed to learn how to be with people her own age.

And she was so curious and bright. Orientation and an interview with the teacher suggested she was intellectually ready and personally able to cope, and she really, really wanted to go; to be with her big brother and sister.

Once again, I had to go through the physical pain of separation. Nicola was OK and fortunately her teacher was lovely, but I was a mess. Two days after she began, she was done with kindergarten and wanted to go to big school with Gabe and Grace. Children are present; they don't realise that going to school means going all day, every day; leaving mum and the life we had lead together.

While she was at school, she engaged with both students and the material, and seemed to be enjoying it, but between the hours of school finishing and school starting we were both in pain (both physical and emotional). Her separation anxiety was expressing itself in stomach pain, sleeplessness and neediness; mine was physically expressed in fatigue and emotionally expressed in emptiness.

My inner voice was still telling me this was the right course of action but I was on the verge of changing my mind until two other aspects of our family life changed.

One of my students arrived for her class and spent the entire class detailing the shortcomings of doing an academic program in a small country school. Gabe was sitting next to us listening and saying nothing. After a massage and relaxation my student left and Gabe came straight into the kitchen while I was cooking dinner.

"I have to go into Canberra for year 11&12".

His plea was impassioned, deep and still; there was no histrionics, no wailing or whinging, just a clear deep knowing that he needed to move on. Grace had already made her case for moving her schooling to Canberra, and Matthew and I knew we had to give them both the opportunity in the 'big smoke'.

Matthew looked at me and said, "Well, you'll just have to take them all in, then".

I guess so ... but I was in shock. Of course, further discussions were had and conditions were made but somehow another major decision in our lives had just been made; another line in the sand. How can life change so quickly?

Through this time my mother had been living with us while my siblings in Sydney found somewhere for her to live. Living independently had become increasingly difficult since my father passed and now had become impossible.

Care was constant and every day her need to move into a care facility was broached. I wanted to nurture her towards acknowledging the reality of her situation but it required so much tenderness and awareness that sometimes I fear I resorted to bullying.

Sorry mum.

In the way of my life over the last few years, all of these aspects of my life converged on the one week. My siblings found a place for my mother and she was able to move in within a week; my son found a program at a Canberra college and they were having an open night in the same week; and it was my sister's birthday in Sydney.

A day of shopping in Canberra for the linen required for my mother's new bed, and we were ready. I would have to drive up to Sydney on the Sunday afternoon, with Nicola and mum, go to my sister's birthday party in the city on the Sunday night, move mum into her new home on the Monday and return home on Tuesday to take Gabe to the open night on the Tuesday night. Easy!

All the way to Sydney I chanted, pranayamed (yogic breathing) and visualised, while talking to mum and keeping Nicola happy. We arrived at my mother's house in Sydney just in time to catch a cab into the city for my sister's birthday. It was a lovely cocktail party but I just didn't feel quite present.

Then it was back to my mother's house and the worse night's sleep since 'curing' insomnia with yoga. Mum was restless, there were sirens, and I was hot and so scared about what I was doing the next day, so I visualised and breathed … for hours. I 'woke' in the morning feeling remarkably serene and energised. Thank God for yoga.

Nicola, mum and I packed up and off we went, me breathing to keep calm. The day consisted of moving my mother in and meeting with staff, reassuring her and spending some time with one of my brothers. Nicola was so beautiful and calm through the whole day. Perhaps it was the time she had spent with my illness or perhaps just some innate understanding that this wasn't about her, but whatever it was, her maturity and patience on that day will forever be in my mind as a testament of the love children are capable of.

Finally, we had to leave and I felt bereft; again the feeling of leaving someone I loved washed over me and I wondered if I was doing the right thing.

I headed back to mum's, exhausted and hardly able to stay awake enough to feed Nicola and myself. Needing to find some paperwork i went into her study. As I looked through her papers I got an insight into the increasing confusion of her mind and I realised we were doing the right thing; it was time to let go.

The next day we returned to my mother to find her knitting and laughing with the other residents. Phew! Now we could go back to Braidwood, and so we left with me silently chanting for the three-hour drive. We arrived home in time for a quick break and to load the rest of the family into the car for the drive to Canberra for the open night.

Yes! Yes! Yes! This was the program Gabe wanted, and Grace also fell for the college system and the same program at the intermediate level. So on the same night we found college for Gabe and a school for Grace, and confirmation we were coming into Canberra.

And the next day Nicola returned to school, a little older and ready to embrace her new life. We had the occasional mental health day and of course late days but not the separation anxiety we had experienced in the previous weeks. With a little sadness, I realised my youngest daughter was on her own way.

Students

I continued tutoring maths students in the afternoon after school and also running a free study group on Saturdays. Most afternoons I had at least one student, sometimes two and at exam times, at least two doubled up for extra preparation.

The study group was run in the local library so that senior students could gather and support each other through the HSC. My role was to help with study technique and provide adult supervision. We did some yoga or relaxation, brought food and generally created an atmosphere of relaxed conscientiousness.

So much was done in those two hours each week and some of it was an exchange of ideas, some of it was support, and it made such a difference to the commitment of those students to establish an enjoyable study routine.

Books

The books that were having the most influence on me during this period were the *Dru Baghavad Gita* and the *Secret Power of Light* by the founder of Dru, Dr Mansukh Patel. Over the summer, I had read *The Journey,* by Brandon Bays, *The Power of Now,* by Eckhardt Tolle and Petrea King's story of her journey with cancer and beyond, and they had all had an impact on my perceptions of my situation, but it was these two books that were providing the material for the deepening of my practice.

The first volume of the Dru Gita, the first six chapters, had been given to me by my first Dru teacher in 2006. I had been reading it for 18 months and now felt ready to graduate to the next two volumes. As with the first volume, I started by reading through then started to open it randomly and read the verses on the page in front of me.

Opening the Gita started to become a practice I eagerly anticipated each day, like calling a good friend for advice. Somehow, the wisdom between the covers came alive and interacted with my life and whatever my challenges were on that day.

Initially I held the books for what seemed like ages and angsted about choosing the right page. My love of the Gita was becoming another source of stress. Then I realised how silly I was being and just trusted that whatever I read, I would learn from. What a relief! I could relax and just trust. Once again the Gita came alive and is still a source of wisdom for me, still like a beloved old friend.

The *Secret Power of Light* talks about the World Peace Flame, the development of Dru Worldwide and the practice of Dru. There were many magic moments when I read about things I had personally experienced or ideas I had thought for a long time; I felt a natural belonging within the philosophy of Dru I had not felt before.

The two moments I remember most were reading about Mansukh's meditation with the flame and his mother's words about the Gayatri mantra. The flame had become Mansukh's friend during his undergraduate years at Bangor University. I had already started to light a flame in the evening with my practice but I yearned to sit with it in the same way as Mansukh.

The Gayatri is the mother of all mantras, evoking the power of light. The Sanskrit was reprinted on the page and for some reason I wanted to learn it. Every day I repeated it over and over again, and it felt so good. I started to repeat it in my mind through the day when I was walking or practicing or cooking.

Then one day I found a recorded version on a bargain cassette I had bought at a sound workshop the year before, and began singing. It lifted my spirits immediately, so I sung it all the time.

One day I was walking through the bush on our land at Majors Creek and began to sing the Gayatri; Nicola began to dance. All through the bush, Nicola danced like a wood nymph while I sang the Gayatri. It was beautiful and Nicola loved it.

My practice

So, now every night I sat with the flame and chanted Nicola to sleep with the Gayatri, then in the morning sat with the flame again and read the Gita. It was simple and moving, and definitely for me. My mind was opened, and the sense of peace I gained began and ended my day.

I continued to visualise and practice yoga, and listened to Chakra Dharanam but increasingly my own meditation practice over took the gentle tones of Chris.

My chakra assignment had also taken on the form of a practice. As I read about, wrote and finally drew each major chakra, I felt like I was becoming attuned to those levels of my being and developing a deeper understanding of the subtle layers of myself.

And a persistent whisper arose in meditation, "Meditation Teacher Training".

Maidenhair Fern, Pap Smear and the Skin Spot

I have never been a gardener but I have a Maidenhead Fern and a Peace Lily that I love with a passion. Perhaps I love them both so much because they were a Christmas gift from my husband; perhaps also because I saved them, particularly the Maidenhair, from near death.

This devotion comes in the form of lavish attention: talking, kissing, caressing and regular watering. As a consequence, they both flourished and became verdant. I can feel the being in the plant; I can feel the life force respond to mine. I have never been this ooby-gooby before.

However, the maidenhair started to change. First it was white on the odd frond. Then excessive amounts of white clingy stuff a bit like spider web began to appear. It was getting worse and my beautiful maiden-hair was starting to look sick.

Every time I looked at her I thought I should go to the nursery in town and ask them about what I could do but for some reason I continued to put it off. I'd noticed that I started to pay her less attention. In fact, I believe I had started to avoid her. Why?

When looking at her the other day I realised the reason I avoided her is because I felt guilty for not looking after her better. Did I love the plant any less? No. Facing her would be facing my own negligence so I avoided it, pretending I am too busy. Are we ever really too busy to love? Even if we have to face our own shortcomings to do so, we are never too busy to love. Once again I am shown the true meaning of unconditional love.

Why is it that human beings, when confronted with an issue in their being in need of nurturing, choose to ignore, do the opposite or deny?

I know you're there, meditation, stillness … maidenhair, Pap smear, skin cancer.

Almost twelve months after I had the first inkling to have a pap smear, the same inkling returned. I had been ignoring it in the same way I had been ignoring my Maidenhair, deliberately avoiding any train of thought that might lead to my cervix. Unfortunately when one meditates regularly such obstinacies can only be sustained for so long before the voice you can't ignore shouts in the middle of stillness. "MAIDEN-HAIR, PAP SMEAR, SKIN CANCER!"

The following day I made an appointment with my GP to have a pap smear, have a skin spot checked and, yes, I started to look after the maidenhair.

The skin spot was one I had asked the doctor to look at a couple of times but it hadn't gone away and it looked a little different. The doctor agreed to remove it and an appointment was made. The procedure was straight forward but the local knocked me around and took away some of the progress I had made. I made it home but only after a rest at the surgery, and very, very slowly.

The pathology returned and sure enough it was precancerous but it was all removed and there was no danger. Once again, I had reason to thank the voice in meditation.

Unfortunately, I had another reason to thank the voice; the Pap smear was also positive for middle grade cell change. Bugger! I only just managed to keep it together for the nurse who had rung to tell me and make another appointment.

I rang my sister and said, "I know there's no point in being angry and I know there's no such thing as 'not fair' but I'm really pissed off and it's not fair!" I couldn't believe it. I knew it wasn't that serious and I knew I would be alright but it was another thing I had to deal with; another thing I had to find a way to accept and live around.

Another colposcopy. Yes more cells but not nearly as bad. No surprise we didn't get it all last year because the mass was so large. Good Oh. At least this can be done with a local and I only had to wait a couple of months.

Oh, and the maidenhair flourished once again.

EBR3, The Seat of Compassion and the Bhajans – Module 4

MARCH 2008

I walked into Module 4 without my wheelchair or sticks (I had taken them with me just in case but left them at the hostel).

Anglicare was again funding my accommodation and transport to and from Canberra but I didn't need to stay at the venue anymore so I booked cheaper accommodation at the youth hostel. A morning and evening ritual began during this time, embedding a beautiful friendship that has given me so much laughter and love.

When I booked my accommodation, transport to and from the venue hadn't occurred to me. In the previous modules a group from the module had been staying at the same place so I assumed I could get a lift.

Wrong. There were only a few people staying at the hostel and they were all walking to the venue.

Walking?!

I could catch a taxi, I could catch a bus if I knew where to stand … or I could walk. If I walked, it would be the longest distance since before I was pregnant with Nicola.

I used to love walking as a mode of transport; walking an hour to school rather than catching the bus, going to uni and later from Annandale to Darlinghurst and back for work. It was meditative and relaxing, and one of the things I missed most when I started to lose my legs.

I would frequently use walking as a temper neutraliser and that's something I really missed. Once I tried to 'walk' off my temper in my power chair and there was nothing satisfying about powering off into the sunset, other than moving independently.

If I pulled this off, it would be gobsmacking … oh well, why not? I can always stop along the way; I can always get a cab if I need to or maybe even a bus.

We set off early because I had no idea how long it would take for me to walk that far. Ten minutes into the journey and we stopped for fresh juices. What a relief. When we started again, I tried to keep up with my friends (pride) but my right side started to go off line and I knew that if I kept that pace there would be no way I could make it all the way.

'Walk to the beat of your heart', and I slowed down to a pace that felt right for me. The others walked on, with the exception of the woman who has since become my confidante and one of my closest friends in the world.

We walked at a very leisurely pace and chatted the whole way. We didn't talk about me or MS or yoga (oh, a little bit about me and a little bit about yoga). We mostly talked about Sharron and her life and children and books. I remember that walk and all similar walks we did through the three modules we stayed at the YHA together with the kind of Vaseline glow usually reserved for the lead actresses in B-grade Hollywood movies.

Even writing about it now, I still don't believe I did it. It was so far! We just kept walking and walking and walking, but as long as I kept that mindful approach to my speed and my step length, I could keep going. The steps were very small by the end and my feet were barely leaving the ground but I made it.

When I arrived there were a few comments about my testimonial, which had now been published in the newsletter but I didn't notice them so much then; I had just walked to the venue and I wanted to do some yoga.

The postures in Module 4 were all strong postures, stimulating the lower chakras i.e. shifting issues of safety and emotional turbulence up into the heart to be transformed. Eka pada ada ada ada … (so don't get Sanskrit names), for example, is a beautiful and regal posture otherwise known as the Mast and involves opening the pelvic girdle (home to the base and second chakra), lifting stuck energy out of the lower spine then twisting it up into an open chest and out through open arms. Awesome!

The three most significant things I remember about that module (aside from the walks) were EBR3, the Seat of Compassion and bhajans, but mostly, the Seat of Compassion.

The Seat of Compassion incorporates four strong postures and a powerful spiral in a challenging and transformative sequence. First we learnt the individual postures we didn't already know and revised those we did know; Chair of the Heart, Charity, Crane and the Seat of Compassion.

Each day I felt stronger as we walked from the YHA and I combined visualising with physical yoga. The key to the balancing postures like the crane was to centre myself somewhere between my navel and pubic bone then move into the posture from this centre.

I still felt like I had little strength or stamina so I let the energy of my body and breath move my limbs and, when in the full posture, I would relax. This is what I had learned from the Dancer in the previous module; to just relax and trust that 'other' layer of my system to hold the posture.

This is hard to explain intellectually because it is not an intellectual thing. It was unfamiliar to the part of me that taught maths and chemistry but increasingly familiar to the part of me that relied on my mind to move energy around my body and keep me upright when the muscles alone weren't going to do it.

There was, and still is, a column of energy that

runs from the base of my spine through and out of my crown, that could with concentration (emphasis on concentration) be moved and balanced depending on the needs of my body.

Each posture was an exercise in concentration, moving into meditation when I found the still point; the point of surrender and trust.

To learn the Seat of Compassion we were split into two groups and each group learned only one half of the sequence. Then we came together in pairs to teach each other the half we had learned; I taught my partner the first half and he taught me the second half, on one side, and then we did the same thing for the other side.

Then we practiced the whole sequence through. Oh my god!

Without much thought, I began the Seat of Compassion. The heart of the sequence is the Seat of Compassion posture; the centre around which the sequence revolves. Every time I have practiced this sequence since, the Dru point when mind, body and spirit merge occurs in this heart…but not on that day.

On that day I was in the resting position at the end of the Charity pose (see **Charity pose and Spinal wave** p238), completely bent over my right leg, balancing with my hands behind my back in prayer position when time stopped and I entered into a different reality.

I suddenly realised how far I had come. Six months ago I had spent most of my time in an electric wheelchair and here I was 'resting' in the charity pose. In that moment, anything was possible. Again I felt invincible.

Tears welled in my eyes.

I finished the rest of the sequence in a surreal non-reality; time slowed and I felt every movement of energy and muscles with the deepest intention. When we completed the spiral at the end of the sequence and came down into the pose of the child, I let go.

The tears, emotion and energy ran wild. There was not a specific thought or emotion that formed the sobs that racked my body, just the magnitude of my journey. The woman nearest me enveloped me as I released (we are now close friends), then my peers stroked and hugged me with such tenderness and love as they passed on their way to a break. Thank you.

One woman, whose friendship I still deeply value, said, "What a journey you have in front of you". It was like she had seen through the gap that had been made in my present into a future I could not imagine. I was too gobsmacked with the journey that had been and where it had brought me to that point.

Another before and after moment.

And bhajans, the yogi version of a party. The increased support for public choirs over the last twenty years demonstrates the yearning and benefits of people singing together; you know, many voices into one, rivers into an ocean, the result of the whole being greater than the sum of its parts etc.

Again and again through my life, I have returned to singing in choirs and groups to experience this sense of sharing something sacred, yet haven't found the avenue that has felt really authentic for me.

Singing bhajans in a group is the yogic version of a public choir. My first experience of this was utterly joyous on the same day as Seat of Compassion. I was intimately aware of the physical progress I had made, as well as the beginnings of feeling part of a wider community, and I was ready to party!

Sitting in the teaching room that evening with all the people who had been part of the day of realisation, singing beautiful Sanskrit chants, galvanised the feeling of community and embedded the feeling of rising above my own limits to find a freedom I hadn't imagined. We sang and danced for an eternity (probably about two hours) then I walked 'home' with my beloved yoga buddy.

Since that night, singing bhajans has remained a source of heightened awareness and an understanding of the love and joy we can share in community. Virtuosity is not the issue; being part of something bigger than yourself is.

EBR3 is a deceptively powerful sequence; quite literally a pump for the heart. When I learned the sequence during module I enjoyed it but it didn't have the physical strength of EBR2 or the foundation essence of EBR1. It wasn't until I started practicing it at home that this wish fulfilling energy block release sequence came into its own for me. (see **EBR3** *p.*239)

Charity pose and Spinal wave

In the Charity pose in the Seat of Compassion we gradually bend over our front foot in a series of waves, pumping the energy from the base of our spine into our open heart, finally resting at our lowest position; relaxing into this position and allowing gravity to stretch out our back, stretching the hamstring, the lower back is lengthening and stimulating the lower chakras to release stuck energy.

The posture begins with my hands behind my heart in Namaste (prayer position), legs in wide stance with core stability strong, hips turned to face over my right leg; pivoting from my hips and keeping table-top back (straight back), I bend over my right leg; first about a quarter of the way, then bending the right leg, core stability on, press into the right foot and curl my spine upright, lifting my sternum last of all.

*This is called the **spinal wave** and creates a wave of energy up the spine into an open lifted heart and out through the crown. The spinal wave is one of my favourite singular movements in Dru because it feels like it is cleansing, energising and balancing my spine in one go; and it can be done sitting, standing, lying visualising or subtly anywhere. For me It is one of the most versatile and useful movements in Dru.*

EBR3

In EBR3, we spend half the first half of the sequence opening our heart and lungs, seeing our higher self reflected back to us and expanding our self esteem with movements that rhythmically expand our chest in all directions and gently twist our spine. Then, when we set our goal in the Archer we can be sure our it will be for the highest good, before sending a thunderbolt of energy behind it in Runner-into-thunderbolt.

I think EBR3 took longer to land because I was still feeling sceptical about some of the more ooby-gooby aspects of Dru but when I practiced it myself I felt transformed by its subtle power; and when I taught it, I watched the most sceptical of students rise to EBR3, and another manifest her goals.

I no longer doubt the hidden power of this sequence.

The Whisper
That Became a Roar –
Meditation Teacher Training

FEBRUARY – APRIL 2008

The whisper that began in January became a roar through February.

My teachers gave me a series of questions to ponder while listening to the roar. Money, family, time and health; practical questions about how I would fit another course into my life. However the bigger questions were personal and I was asking them of myself.

From the experience of my life in the previous few years I had learned that the pragmatics of life seem to expand or contract depending on what is being demanded of them. There was this strange feeling of testing fate; if I was meant to do the meditation teacher training, I would be able to, somehow.

Why did I want to do the course? A friend asked what I was trying to prove. She may have been playing devil's advocate or she may have been posing a genuine question (I still don't know). Regardless it was an interesting thing to ponder. Was I trying to prove anything and if so, what and why?

I returned to my meditation practice for the answer to that question. I looked carefully through what had become a yearning to do the meditation teacher training and I couldn't find any evidence of pride or ego, just that now familiar deep pull and some disconcerting fear. Where does the fear come from? Once again, I sat with it for a few days while I searched my waking intellect. A conversation with another friend elucidated one aspect of the fear – the possibility of losing my instinctual love of meditation.

My practice had grown out of my love for sitting in stillness with the flame and 'accidents' of peace and stillness before Dru; I didn't want it to become a chore or an intellectual exercise. I loved meditation and I didn't want to lose it. That fear was almost enough to stop me from doing the course.

The course blurb boasted a rigorous study of the process and science of meditation and … well I didn't really care; I didn't want to study, I just really wanted to do it. This inner conflict remained unresolved and to some extent still is; the balance between learned knowledge and innate or intuitive wisdom is one I continue to explore.

This still left a hidden fragment of inner conflict. Back to the flame. This deeper source of fear remained elusive, hiding behind comfort and my identity as mother and my perceptions of my family's needs.

A one-on-one with a Buddhist spiritual teacher in 1998 began with him asking what I was worried about. Was it that obvious? Since leaving my children two days before, I had felt constant anxiety about their wellbeing. The angst prevented me from fully engaging in the weekend.

In reality, the children were fine; they were with my husband and I trusted him completely to care for them and love them. So what was the problem?

The problem was with me and my attachment to my identity as a parent. I felt that not being with my children 24/7 meant I was neglecting them and using the associated anxiety to prevent me from fully engaging in the weekend. I was standing on the edge looking in, as I had always done; perhaps even using my mother-anxiety to avoid engaging.

Of course, underneath I knew because as soon as the master said "they are fine", I knew he was right and instantly surrendered. What followed was amazing and began my journey with meditation.

This was the moment I returned to when looking at this last fragment of fear regarding the meditation teacher training. In essence I was afraid of losing my identity as a devoted parent.

I think what I realised at that moment was that the job of devoted parent was ensuring one's children were cared for and loved; it wasn't necessarily to be there 24 hours a day, wiping every nose leek or pooey bottom. Other people, e.g. my husband, can look after my children as well as I can.

When I checked back with the flame, repeatedly, the answer was the same: the children will be fine. But still the fear was present.

Back to the flame to find the next layer. How do people cope without spending time knowing these layers?

The real fear was of change; by doing meditation teacher training I would somehow begin a process that would take me away from the comfort of everything I knew, and of course, my beloved family.

In the light of meditation, the answer was, yes, there would be change but that this change would ultimately result in closer relationships not distancing. So now I knew what I was afraid of but not why I wanted to do the course. Unlike the yoga teacher training, I didn't particularly want to be a meditation teacher, so that wasn't why.

The answer came through a conversation with my husband. We were talking about communication and I said my goal "was to remove all the blocks in my communication so I could be a completely clear vessel and I wasn't going to stop until my last breath".

Wow. It was one of those sentences that just came out without pre-meditation but once it's out the truth is undeniable and it hangs in the air between you as if to engrave its truth in your mind in a way that can never be wiped from the record. That's why I want to do the meditation teacher training.

I went back to the flame and found harmony, and made my decision. This deep yearning was stronger and louder than the fears and pragmatics combined. In the face of this certainty, the 'why nots' laid down their arms and surrendered. So I wrote my letter of application to my teachers and they welcomed me into the course.

Then I set about getting funding. I was lucky to find two government funding sources to begin the course; accommodation and transport to Canberra once again came from Anglicare; and with permission from my teachers, I was on my way with only weeks to spare – plenty of time.

I arrived feeling very inexperienced and very anonymous. Everyone seemed to know each other and I hardly knew anyone. Yet I also felt incredible relief with the lack of recognition. There were three other people from my yoga teacher training group and a couple of members of the support crew from the three modules so maybe I could just sit on the edge.

In the first couple of days there were a few people who quietly and discretely asked me if I was the person in the newsletter, telling me my story was inspiring and that they had told their classes. That was nice, a little embarrassing, but nice. My ego was flattered in a strange and not entirely comfortable way.

Then on the third day in a small group exercise, one of the other participants discovered it was me who was in the newsletter and was astonished by how well I was. Like many people who read the story, it was assumed I would be well but not *well and agile*. That was it, it was out.

Again, it is hard to describe the effect this has on

the way people relate to me and also the effect it has on me, personally. It was quite a confusing blend of appeasing an injured ego and creating a new identity; embarrassing because I felt/feel like what I did was ordinary and I was/am ordinary; and gratifying to see how much people were inspired by my story. In essence, I didn't really know what to say, so I smiled a lot and said thank you.

That aside, the module was awesome. Over six modules we were going to explore the layers of our being with meditation and learn how to teach. In yogic terms, layers of our being meant the five koshas, the physical layer, the energetic layer, the layer of our motivations, the layer of belief and connection, and finally the layer of bliss. An in-depth exploration of who we are.

The first layer was physical, so we spent four days yoga-ing, relaxing and learning the basic technique that would take us through the course. It was fantastic to spend such a long time in silence, getting to know our body.

Another set of practices to fit into my life.

Walking to the Beat of My Heart, Part 2

APRIL 2008

One day while walking Nicola to school in our daily ritual of being slightly late, as we travelled that same street into town that had become my favourite stretch of footpath in the world, I realised I was rushing again. Not only was I rushing but my right side was in the process of going off line and I was feeling stressed.

My gait had become lurching as I forced my steps into longer strides, my right leg was giving way every few steps and I was in danger of losing my balance; I was lifting my hip to get my foot off the ground and my spine was leaning forward as if I was leading with my chin… I was leading with my chin.

Why?

Nicola was four, in kindergarten. The world wasn't going to stop spinning if the four-year-old misses the first few minutes of the day, yet I felt external pressure to meet some hypothetical standard of perfect behaviour. I was walking to someone else's beat and it was costing me my physical function and mental calm. Not to mention the calm of the four-year-old – poor Nicola was puffing and panting trying to keep up with me.

So, finally I stopped and realigned my body into Tadasana, the mountain pose, and began to walk with this awareness, allowing my feet to fall where it felt natural for them to fall. Again, I had the feeling that someone was holding my skeleton from a golden cord through my spine and coming out of the crown of my head.

All of my muscles and ligaments seemed to relax and my bones fell where they should fall, all the way down to my feet. Walking became effortless; my step lengths were much shorter than what I had been trying to achieve but felt much more natural. The back of my neck was long and my crown was pointing straight up; rather than leading with my chin I was now leading with my heart.

Again, it occurred to me how much time and energy I had spent through my life, trying to keep up with people; trying to match their speed when my legs and body were shorter, and how much energy it cost me.

This revolutionised the way I moved, particularly walking. Sometimes I had the stretch to walk with longer strides and sometimes I had 'lollypop' steps, and sometimes a shuffle but, if I walked with what I had, whatever that was, I would always get there in much better condition.

Of course I still forget sometimes and find myself walking to someone else's beat but when I realise, usually by feeling MS symptoms, re-alignment and my own beat are just a breath away.

Oh, and we did get to school in a much more pleasant fashion, with four-year-old smiling and chatting rather than puffing and panting.

Back to The Classroom

After I left hospital in 2004 and was not allowed back into the school where I had been teaching, I thought my days in the classroom were over. I wasn't a career teacher or think I was the most brilliant teacher in the world, and I wasn't sure I even wanted to be a classroom teacher; I just loved watching the transformation that can occur in teenagers over a period of time.

My professional skills had been improved so much by my experience in Britain, I felt like I had been cut off from a career path before I had had the chance to really explore it fully. And of course, the exacerbation in 2006 reinforced that feeling of loss.

What was I going to do for the rest of my life? What was I here for? Was all that tutoring and teacher training a waste?

Then at the beginning of the school term 2008, I re-registered with the education department as a casual teacher, thinking a couple of days a week at the local school would be good; "maybe I *could* do it again". Within weeks I was offered a temporary full-time position for six weeks, replacing a teacher on extended leave teaching maths and one class of science.

No-one, least of all me, knew if I could carry a full-time load with yoga and meditation practice and study, parenting and my continuing maths students, as well as study group, but there was only one way to find out.

On the first day, one of the executive was very clear about the need to inform her if I felt any return of symptoms. I knew what that meant from my experience in the UK, and that as much as anything else made me determined to make it, even if it meant the odd bit of faking it. I simply set my intention at succeeding with complete stubborn denial of any other possibility.

Soon after the meditation module I went back into the classroom. It was quite confronting to once again be standing in front of a classroom of teenagers, trying to impart at least a modicum of mathematical knowledge. I felt nervous, out of practice.

"Maybe I've lost it, if I ever had it."

I reverted to what had become normal, I did yoga in my mind; this was becoming my natural response to any situation. Whenever I had the opportunity in a pause between classes, on the way to class, at lunchtime or even in the quiet moments during class (although there weren't many of these opportunities), I would practice yoga.

I still had an 'all-day' practice but now it was fitted in between the cracks of work and family. It was a motley combination of practices from Module 4 of the Yoga Teacher Training and Module 1 of the Meditation Teacher Training.

I began to practice meditation with my eyes open so I could practice the meditation exercises we had learned through the module. In my morning and evening meditation practice at home I followed the guidelines more closely, but during the day I explored the possibilities of meditation in life.

What I re-discovered was that I could maintain an altered state of consciousness all day, in varying degrees, by doing the smallest practices, constantly. I had discovered this the first time after Module 1 when I visualised, relaxed and meditated constantly to relieve the madness, but had lost the impetus a little with recovery.

When I started teaching again I found I needed to rediscover constant practice to keep functioning. Whenever I felt the fatigue of MS or another symptom appear I would simply find a practice I could do either in my head or unobtrusively, and my awareness (and quite often my physical state) would change quite quickly.

I visualised sequences and postures from Module 4 when I had the time and space to concentrate but mostly I did smaller practices that could be done in a few minutes while walking around.; for example parts of EBR1 like the Arm Rotations (see *Arm Rotations* p.256), which I had been doing since learning them in Module 1. On the surface a seemingly simple practice but profound in its effect of opening up the heart and gently working the muscles of the shoulder girdle, while gently massaging that space between the shoulder blades that's really difficult in any other way.

I also discovered the value of Pranayama, the yogic art of moving energy around the body using the breath, because pranayama is an easy practice while walking or sitting in the staffroom, and nobody notices you are doing anything (not unlike visualisation).

I had always thought I was crap at Pranayama because I had been asthmatic and my confidence in my breath was limited, and MS had also limited my stamina in repetition of breathing exercises and at times my muscular ability.

However, during this period I learnt that like all practices, Pranayama could be modified to suit the practitioner, and also, like all practices, overdoing it hurts – sometimes less is more – and, most importantly, sometimes making the slightest alteration to my breathing is enough to change my consciousness. The effect was that I was walking around in everyday life, functioning and relating in a state of altered consciousness. (see **Pranayama** p.257)

In 2007 I visualised constantly to transcend the difficulties of my circumstances – to feel peace – and the by-product was physical function. Yet somewhere during my recovery I lost that focus. The return to physical function was so overwhelming I forgot some of the most important lessons of the journey.

So, just less than 12 months later when I went

back into the classroom I had to re-learn the value of constant practice but this time the goals and benefits were reversed. This time I was practicing to keep functioning, physically and the by-product was peace.

How amazing to be working in a high school, and feeling calm and peaceful; to be parenting, working, tutoring and practicing, with a chronic illness, and feeling calm and peaceful.

When I reflect now I realise the hours of practice I did while working gave me a sense of stillness so the action of working in the world originated in stillness. There was no need to use excess energy in being busy because I could just act when I needed and leave the rest.

Mornings, getting out the door, are of course exceptions to any rules of equanimity and should be declared a universal disaster zone for spiritual or even reasonable awakening – anyone reading this who has ever tried to get three children, themselves and a husband out the door every morning with vaguely clean clothes, (vaguely resembling school uniform or perhaps not even vaguely), with edible lunches in their bags and some kind of writing device in their pocket will know what I mean.

And well, I am simply not a domestic goddess.

Arm Rotations.

- *Begin by tucking your tailbone under and allowing the curving movement to move up the spine to the crown, creating a wave of energy up through your torso and resulting in your spine curled.*

- *Then tilt your pelvis back and allow that movement to flow up the spine, lifting your sternum at the end, opening your chest; again resulting in a wave of energy through your spine.*

- *Breathe out as you curl your spine and breathe in as you open your chest.*

- *Repeat a few times to establish the spinal wave.*

- *Then on the breath in, and with your arms a little distance away from your sides, allow the movement to flow down your arms into your elbows and wrists, and rotate your palms forward as your chest opens.*

- *On the breath out, the movement flows down your arms and you rotate your arms backwards.*

- *Continue the rotations, gradually raising the arms to shoulder height.*

- *Rotate the arms in alternate directions so that one arm rolls forwards at the same time as the other one rolls backwards, maintaining the spinal wave as you alternate.*

- *Your head turns in the direction of the up-*

turned hand and perhaps visualise a ball of light or affirmation to roll from one hand to another. I find the point of stillness in my heart and let my mind rest there, so the movement originates from the stillness.

- *Lower your arms to your side when you are ready.*

Whenever I do this movement I feel like my heart is being given a massage while opening and relaxing the entire shoulder girdle, and while I was teaching I needed as much heart opening as possible!

Pranayama

Pranayama is the yogic science of moving energy around the body and altering consciousness with the breath. Changing our breathing pattern is the quickest and easiest way of changing our state of mind. It is also very powerful and needs to be approached with some caution.

For me the essence of Pranayama is peace of mind, regardless of the specific practice.

- *Changing your breathing cycle can be a powerful practice so be aware of the feelings in your mind and body;*
- *If you begin to feel any unpleasant sensations, such as tingles, light-headedness or giddiness return to normal breathing, lie down on your stomach or go and so something soothing and*

relaxing – ALWAYS LISTEN TO THE LIMITS OF YOUR OWN BODY; and

- *If you have a heart condition or blood pressure issues, don't breathe too deeply and don't hold the breath.*

Deep Yogic Breath (DYB) *is the foundation of most Pranayama exercises and as a practice on its own generates fuller breath and a deep sense of calm.*

- *If you are sitting on a chair, ensure your feet are flat on the floor or solid surface (telephone books make great foot stools for breathing practice), your lower legs are at right angles with your thighs and thighs are at right angles with your back.*

- *If you are on the floor, try a cushion under the rear of your buttocks to ensure the pelvis is tilted slightly forward to give a slight arch in the lower back.*

- *Whether on the floor or a chair, engage core stability and become aware of your straight spine, roll back each shoulder and notice your head sitting on top of your neck.*

- *Now, take a few breaths to allow your body to relax into this position; allow your gaze to soften.*

- *When you are ready, focus your attention on the muscle at the base of the breast bone that controls your breathing – the diaphragm.*

- *Allow your diaphragm to slowly expand*

down into the abdomen and as you do this, notice your lungs filling with air; contract the diaphragm and the breath leaves the lungs.

- *Repeat this a few times and you may already notice a difference in your mind and body.*
- *Once you are comfortable with this breathing pattern, become aware of the bottom third of your lungs and breathe into and out of this part of your lungs for a few breaths.*
- *Now, become aware of the middle section of your lungs and on your next in-breath, breathe into the bottom then the middle of your lungs (around heart level, otherwise called thoracic), then breathe out from the bottom then middle. Repeat for a few breaths.*
- *For the final stage, become aware of the very top section of your lungs and breathe into the bottom, middle then into this top section of your lungs, allow the air to fill to the collarbones; exhale, again by contracting the diaphragm, from the bottom, middle and then top of your lungs. Repeat this no more than ten times in a session to begin with and gradually build into a longer practice.*
- *Allow your body to relax slowly into this breathing pattern, never straining or breathing to your full capacity.*
- *Take a few moments to ease back into normal breathing and notice how you feel.*

So What Happens
After Class?

So what was the result of all of those hours of practice? Was there a transformative process I was engaging in other than keeping my body functioning, and if so, what was the impact of this on the rest of my life?

The reality of that time, in fact the previous twelve months, was constant transformation of every aspect of how I lived and perceived my life. Many of my habitual patterns of relating and thinking and feeling were being brought up for re-assessment, and if necessary, releasing.

Within a very short time I had moved from being physically disabled to physically functioning and working and this was a huge shift psychologically. It seemed everything was up for negotiation; nothing was a given.

It felt to me like there was no solid place for me to stand.

My children of course were constant, as were my students but even these relationships were being reframed by my growth and my changing physical circumstances. I had no idea where this process would lead and what my future held within that, and I struggled with this new uncertainty. I looked for ways to make sense of the shifting sands of my inner world regarding my future and couldn't.

Hadn't MS already taught me the futility of building castles in the sky of my future? Did I have to learn those lessons all over again?

I experienced such deep fear; every habit I released seemed to take me further away from what I had always known without a clear direction as to where I was going. I feared I was moving away from everything and everyone I knew but there was no going back.

And, of course, even this feeling of uncertainty fluctuated in its intensity. The only true certainty was my intention and my practice. My intention was inner peace, still, and my practice was a mix of visualising and actual physical yoga, and meditation.

I was so over the feeling of madness that had plagued me through my life, and even though it was costing immediate emotional security, this deep yearning to be free was stronger than the fear, and I believed it was possible.

I had heard or read from spiritual teachers and texts that for most of us to really achieve spiritual growth, our yearning to be free of the madness has to be so strong that we will do anything to achieve it; this was where I was at that time. I was done with madness.

Every time I heard my teacher talk about freedom or read about freedom in the Gita or one of the other spiritual texts I was dipping into, I wanted it; not just wanted like one wants a piece of chocolate cake but rather a deep soulful yearning with all my being. I wanted to be free and I was willing to do anything to achieve it and I was not going to stop until I did.

Now, of course, I realise it never stops.

So whenever uncertainty became 'too uncertain' I would come back to the one certainty, me, my centre, my intention and the practice that seemed to be taking me there.

Gradually, over the twelve months since the meditation weekend where I had decided to join the teacher training course, the intention of finding inner peace had become a daily prayer and then, without me realising it, my life became the prayer manifest in material reality.

My intention began my day with my morning practice and became an unspoken component of every aspect of my life; eating, cooking, communicating and teaching.

I Can Feel It!

WINTER 2008

The healing journey can be a delightful journey of discovery. Sometimes it feels like every day there is some incremental change, and at other times weeks will go by where nothing seems to happen and then something amazing will happen.

There were random improvements that seem to come out of nowhere, while other improvements were specifically programmed with my yoga practice and aligned with my menstrual cycle.

An example of the latter was a month where I was working with my lower back and hamstrings. Physically I was experiencing tightness in my hamstrings which limited the length of my paces and the yoga I could do, as well as a tightness and ache in my lower back. Emotionally I was feeling constricted and anxious.

My yoga practice was focussed on hamstring stretches and twisting of my lower back, as well as other postures that moved energy from my lower back to be released. As the month moved towards the full moon, the tension in my body and my emotions built until the cause for my emotional anxiety surfaced, and it felt like my whole being burst like a bubble with the onset of menses.

My practice became minimal over the following week as I rested and when I began again my hamstrings had stretched, my lower back eased and the pain had gone. This pattern of physical symptoms being tied in to emotional issues, linked with my menstrual cycle, became a useful tool and one I still use in my healing journey.

I watch for the physical symptoms and as I get closer to the pre-menstrual phase of my cycle, I watch for the issues causing me (and those around me) grief. I use yoga and meditation to get underneath the surface of the issue and allow that cause to rise, to be released before I release, physically. Then I rest for the time of menses and come out with the physical and emotional symptom relieved.

Of course, there are layers to both physical and emotional issues so I would return again and again to the ongoing issues of my life and at first I would think, "Oh no, not this again, I thought I'd dealt with this", thinking I was failing or going backwards or at the very least standing still. However, each time I returned to the same issue it was at the next layer; like returning to the same point on a spiral but at the next rung down and perhaps seeing another aspect of my life where this habit was expressing itself.

The more random discoveries were the most delightful because they were a surprise. An example of randomness occurred one night eating dinner with one of my more subtle symptoms and my youngest daughter.

One night in winter we were having a picnic on the floor in the lounge room by the fire because that was the only room that was warm. I was sitting next to Nicola who brushed my foot with her hand.

Not a big deal you would think but I felt it.

Losing my sensation of touch was one of the first symptoms I noticed consistently in Britain in 2004; it was like feeling the world through a rubber glove and I loved feeling the world without a rubber glove. The loss and the degree of the loss was patchy through my body, and I felt it (or not) worse on my feet.

My kinaesthetic world had been dulled in this way, increasingly for at least the last four years, and before that in patches for about five years.

"Do that again", I said.

Nicola (and the rest of the family looked at me as If I had just lost yet another sandwich in my already diminished picnic box) but she did it anyway.

"I can feel it," I shouted. "I can feel it! I can feel it! I can feel it!"

I laughed and cried and Nicola kept touching my ankle, feeling very pleased she had done something of such consequence. All night and the next day I mar-velled at how much I could 'suddenly' feel. Maybe it had been happening for a long time and I hadn't noticed it but it seemed like a miracle to me to be able to feel the world again.

Another consequence of the same symptom had been an inability to accurately determine the heat of something – tea cup, water etc. In fact, I was banned from running Nicola's baths or even my own showers because I had scolded her once and myself many times. I had many times scalded myself while cooking or holding/drinking hot cups of tea or using hot water from the tap but only realised afterwards when I saw the scald. My family were repeatedly telling me to "put that down, it's hot".

Over the days and weeks following the ankle touching incident, I started to notice being scalded. It happened many times a day. No wonder the tips of my fingers were always red but now I was feeling it. Every time I felt the pain of being scalded I thanked whatever I could feel again.

My sense of touch continued to improve and I scalded myself less and less, but to this day I still am grateful when I feel scalded.

Stillness Is Not My Problem – Action Is

15TH JULY 2008

I had just watched the documentary about Lincoln Hall, the man who survived a night out on Everest in freezing conditions that should have cost him his life, when something hit my consciousness like a well aimed arrow. It was about belief.

Paraphrasing, he said it wasn't enough to think he might live; he had to believe he was going to live. I think it was the same for me in my recovery. Somewhere I had to believe it was possible; that I had some power in this situation, and underneath I did.

As I watched the documentary I also realised it was the meditation retreat 10 years ago that gave me that faith. I have referred to this retreat a couple of times but here is a slightly different aspect.

Since early childhood I have suffered bronchial asthma, including several hospitalisations and steroid dependence. I didn't go anywhere without my Ventolin and rarely went a day without using it. Yet after leaving a two-day Open Way Buddhist meditation retreat near Byron Bay, asthma has not returned as a chronic illness.

In the worst moments of Multiple Sclerosis I have experienced pneumonia and tightness in the chest, for which I have used my puffer, but not since the day of leaving the retreat have I experienced the debilitating everyday chronic illness that is asthma.

Before that weekend I had entertained the possibility of self-healing through the mind but it wasn't until weeks turned into months then into years between Ventolin doses that I really believed it was possible; that I could actually do it myself.

I remember the moment. I had been meditating and yoga-ing for one and a half days, in silence, the yoga clearing the energy blocks in my body and the meditation clearing my mind, when I sat with Hogensen. A moment came when the space between us filled with a beautiful light and I felt like I was coming home, a spiritual coming home and then it was gone. I hadn't experienced anything like that before, neither have I since.

I have held onto this memory ever since, hoping that I would have that experience again but now I realise I can let it go and learn the lesson. The lesson was that the mind has the power. The memory was always there, available to me.

Lincoln Hall had been meditating for years and had

the power of meditation to navigate the challenges of mountain climbing and his life. When it came to this crisis he had the skill to use the power of his mind.

It was the same for me when I started the yoga course and is the same now. I knew I could find peace in chaos and the healing effect that could have because I had lived it, was still living it.

I didn't need to read a book about spiritual healing or be convinced of the connection between spirit and physical wellbeing because in the naivety of ignorance I had experienced it for myself. In evidence based medicine, I was my own evidence.

I didn't have to think it might be and I didn't need to have faith.

For me, yoga and meditation was the key to unlocking that door to peace and still is.

LLETS As
Performance Art

For the previous few months thought of the errant cells that had resurfaced on my cervix had been pushed to the back of my mind while retaining a slight presence.

Finally the date for my LLETS procedure came around and I could allow them to come centre stage. Little did I know I would also be centre-stage.

It had been decided that because I had done all this before that it was a good opportunity to demonstrate a LLETS procedure to a few medical students. I didn't mind, did I? I guess not.

So there I was in stirrups with a light being shone where a light wasn't meant to shine, and an audience of three, the operating gynaecologist and the attending nurse (who was absolutely fabulous, as was the doctor). Thank God for meditation.

I controlled my breathing and deeply relaxed my body and mind, peace descended, and a LLETS procedure as performance art became an opportunity to practice surrender.

I know this will seem strange but despite the pain that followed (and whoever says LLETS procedures don't hurt are male) and the MS exacerbation that resulted, I felt the same peace of mind I experienced after any extended period of yoga or meditation practice; stillness within chaos, regardless of good or bad.

The Gateway to Living – Module 5

JULY 2008

Module 5 was the gateway to living rather than existing. It was now July and it was becoming clear my recovery was not going anywhere; in fact to the contrary, my condition was continuing to improve. Now I felt some obligation to do something with it and I had no idea what or how or even why.

My psychology was still *existing*, even though I had given back my power chair and cancelled my disability allowance; in my mind I was still disabled.

In the medical crises of my life I had had an ambiguous relationship with death and through my mentoring with Andrew had discovered I was more afraid of living than dying, a little like the mortality version of being more afraid of success than failure (which I have also experienced). So now I needed to learn how to live, like a crawling baby learns how to walk – I think sometimes I still fall.

The reason module 5 was so integral in this process of learning to walk was twofold: firstly I felt like the practices worked on stimulating and unblocking the centre of dynamism and enthusiasm; and secondly it was the interim assessment: our opportunity to sit an assessment that would allow us to teach classes as student-teachers, if we passed.

The practices included the eagle, sitting spinal twist, warrior sequence and the cleansing breath, and as I practiced them over the next few months (and still today), they filled me with a strength and a courage to act as I had never experienced before.

The eagle locks at the base of the spine with legs crossed over and the thoracic spine with our arms crossed over, then builds up energy between using breath with the spinal wave and folding over from the hips. A few breaths in this folded, locked position, enables intense focus and stillness. Then in one graceful and powerful motion, unfold and unblock.

It releases energy into the whole body-mind complex, for me focussing on my dynamism centre and my heart.

Andrew demonstrated this posture in the module and I was in the front row. When he did the dynamic version, the unfolding was so potent that the person next to me screamed and jumped backwards a step and we all gasped. I am sure I wasn't the only person in the room who wanted some of what he had.

The eagle has been with me ever since and whenever I perform this posture I feel such an infusion of power and strength, not to mention clarity and focus.

The sitting spinal twist is a posture I used to do with the television after Romper Room. I loved twisting my body into knots and still do. I first encountered it as an adult in Bellingen with a lovely yoga teacher who encouraged us to move our internal organs around, getting the twist in the lower back.

Learning the Dru version took the posture to a deeper level as I became aware of the twist as it moved up my spine, releasing tension gradually as each vertebra twisted around and the muscles around my spine released. Finally, to rest with my open heart was and remains beautiful. On return there always seems to be a sucking in at the heart.

This posture never ceases to make me feel energised and generous, while bringing a satisfied smile to my face. I have learnt, practice and teach a version of the Sitting Spinal Twist for anywhere you aren't doing yoga (see **Workplace Sitting Spinal Twist** p.279).

The Warrior sequence speaks for itself. Warrior 1, 2 and 3, together or in isolation, never cease to give me courage and strength when I think I have none. Somehow, even if my legs are shaky, I can relax into the warrior and feel strong; and if I am visualising, my posture becomes straighter and my head is held higher.

The cleansing breath just made my brain feel like it was in a brain version of a carwash – I so loved this practice I used to do it all the time when I first learned it (unfortunately perhaps too much as I strained my breathing muscles in the process). However, it did seem to clean my thoughts of some pretty limiting ideas of how I could live.

And, well, the interim assessment was a validation of my practice and my capacity to share this, perhaps more so than approval of my teaching skills.

I arrived at the module realising perhaps I had not done enough technical preparation. I knew the postures intimately and had visualised them, practiced them, read about them and written about them but I hadn't studied them. And vitally, I hadn't practiced teaching them.

After a little cramming with my yoga buddy, I decided to just do what I do in my head, but aloud, and hope for the best. For the second time in the yoga course (and possibly my life), I turned myself inside out and spoke what I had only internalised until then.

It was quite bizarre and feels vaguely pretentious, but strangely it felt comfortable; for those moments of teaching my 'class', I felt like a yoga teacher even though I was just sharing what I did in my head. I got the first glimpse that maybe I could do this.

Over the next few months, I started a small class and began to teach. I had shared bits with my maths students but now I started to actually teach full hour and a half classes.

Workplace Sitting spinal twist

- *Sitting with your buttocks on the edge of your chair and your spine straight and relaxed.*
- *Breathe out and engage core stability*
- *Breathe in and lengthen through your spine, lifting your breastbone and raising your right arm to shoulder height (or your own comfort level)*
- *As you breathe out, cross your left hand over to the outside of your right thigh and begin twisting you lower spine then middle spine to the right until your right arm reaches the back of the chair*
- *Rest as you breathe in*
- *Breathe out and use your arm to lever your upper body around into the twist a little further*
- *If it is comfortable, stay in the twist for a few breaths before returning to the centre on an in-breath.*
- *Repeat to the other side.*

This stretches the muscles of the back, and neck, opening the muscles of the chest, while massaging your abdominal organs and improving digestion. Fab on many fronts!

Meditation Teacher Training – Module 2

The sound of 1000 bells

There is a story about a man who is seeking enlightenment.

He is told if he goes to a particular beach and sits and waits and listens, he will hear the ringing of 1000 bells and become enlightened. The keeper of the bells showed him where to sit.

He sat and he waited, day after day but heard nothing and finally gave up.

He began to walk away from shore but in desperation turned one more time toward the beach, having let go of any hope of hearing the bells. As he looked into the sea and the sky he began to see the beauty of the scene before him, a beauty he had not seen while waiting for the bells.

He became entranced by the beauty, noticing the ripples

becoming waves and coming to rest on the sand; the glinting sparkles as the sunlight danced off the sea; and wisps of white that stretched across the sky, forming and unforming in their impermanence.

His mind became still. All grasping left him and a deep sense of contentment arose in his heart, and from contentment came joy.

He watched for what seemed like an eternity but could have been a moment. Then the faint ringing of a bell came to his ears on the sea breeze. First it was just one soft bell, then another and another. Each began softly, gently increasing in volume, almost imperceptibly until he was surrounded by the chorus of 1000 bells.

Tears streamed down his eyes and his heart was fulfilled. He no longer needed for anything and turned to the keeper in gratitude but the keeper was no longer there – the man had now become the keeper of the bells.

I had heard this story at a previous yoga module and had felt the yearning to hear the thousand bells but when I heard it again at the second meditation teacher training module, another layer of meaning landed.

I was in a meditation just before lunch on the fourth day of the module. I had been waiting for the moment when my world would change but it hadn't. I had worked so hard and gone very deep but nothing had occurred.

I was trying particularly hard – 'it had to happen this time'. We were working with our breath and bandhas (energy blocks), and it felt like I was almost bursting a blood vessel I was trying so hard but it wasn't happening. Finally I stopped trying; maybe it just wasn't going to happen this time. I let go.

Moments later Andrew began telling the 1000 bells story, so beautifully and so eloquently that I was entranced once again. I stopped trying to become enlightened, I stopped trying anything and became completely absorbed in the beauty of Andrew's story-telling.

All of my senses were present and my mind became still. In that moment I heard the faint tinkling of bells, the most beautiful sound I had ever heard. I too wept with joy.

Like the man in the story, it was in my surrender to the moment that the bells lay.

Now I was ready for six months of noticing the flow of energy through my mind–body system.

Migration to the City

JANUARY 2009

I began 2009 with the highest energy levels I had experienced since way before diagnosis, and my mind was focussed on facilitating our move to Canberra.

First stop, finding a house. My friends in Canberra had, almost exclusively, told me horror stories of the rental market in Canberra; waiting lists, outrageous rents and unethical leasing practices. Yet I remained positive – 'there would be a house, we would find a house, we always had before and now was no different'.

However, my first forays into the Canberra rental market were not encouraging. Rentals were at least $50 a week more expensive than when I first began looking six months before, and the area we needed to move into was the catchment area for the most popular high school in Canberra (the same reason we wanted to move into the area) and, unbeknown to us, also one of the most popular primary schools, hence a most sought after residential address i.e. even more expensive.

The first couple of trips were characterised by agents forgetting or mistaking the appointment, or losing houses due to misrepresentation by the agent.

January was hot and MS was present.

Then I thought I would try a Saturday of viewings. At every house there were long queues and applications that wanted the details of birthmarks and any potentially nasty personal habits.

Feeling a little disheartened, I bought the paper and called a Dru friend. The paper yielded a private rental with a viewing in the afternoon and the phone call yielded a much needed debrief with someone who reminded me of the concept of co-creating my reality.

I arrived early for the viewing before anyone arrived and looked around, determined to maximise the possibility of success. After my conversation with my friend, I decided that if this place was clean with standing walls, a toilet and a roof, I would take it if I could. Yep, it ticked all the boxes, it would be fine.

By the time the landlord arrived there were three other interested parties (and by the time I left about half an hour later there were another ten or so looking through the house). I felt like a granny at the January sales, elbows out and ready to stamp on the foot of anyone getting in my way.

I managed to be the first to go in and had a quick look around but had already decided so approached the landlord and explained my circumstances. His children had attended the same school my daughter wanted to and said it was a fantastic school, and took my details. I drove home to Braidwood feeling much calmer and resolved to whatever happened. An hour after returning home he called to offer me the house. Yay! We had a house!

On the following Monday I paid the bond and the first few weeks rent and had a date to move in a couple of weeks. We did it. A nine month lease enabled us the freedom to move if it wasn't working and the security of knowing we had a house. It was no Taj Mahal but we were in Canberra and I felt so grateful. It felt like a castle to me for most of the nine months.

Of course, it hadn't occurred to me that the move might be traumatic. January heat and MS aside, I had managed to intellectually bypass the fact that we were about to separate the family. However, as we began to separate possessions between Canberra-destined and Majors Creek-destined, a deep sadness began to twirl its creepers through my optimism.

I was moving to Canberra under the auspices of furthering our children's education but it felt like we were separating; we were paying independently and organising our separate lives, separately. At times I would just crumble and weep.

We sent the big kids over to Canberra to begin unpacking and stayed in Braidwood with Nicola to finish the last minute packing and cleaning. Each night we stayed at the Creek and each morning we came into town in the morning. Nicola was amazing in her ability to just be in the chaos while we sorted and packed and cleaned.

I chanted through the heat and used a yogic cooling breath (see *Yogic cooling breath* p.60) when it became too much, and stopped when I needed.

I wandered through the house from one job to another. Whenever I couldn't decide what I was going to do next I would just do what was in front of me – 'whatever I do now, I won't have to do tomorrow' – so every decision was the right one and life was calm.

Finally it was done and a week before school started in Canberra, Nicola and I moved to Canberra and Matthew moved to the Creek.

It's funny, we had often talked about living separately and coming together on the weekends, me in the city and Matthew in the country, but I didn't think it would happen so soon, if it ever happened at all.

Cleaning the Toilet *and* Putting the Garbage Out

FEBRUARY 2009

We set up our house as quickly as we could. Gabe and his girlfriend in one room, Grace and Nicola in the second, and a study in the third (Gabe and his girlfriend were both studying and needed the privacy). I had always wanted to just have a futon on the floor that I rolled up every morning and that was my plan – to sleep on the floor of the girls' bedroom.

I didn't get to the futon because the girls' floor was never clear enough and they filled the room so my clothes went into the linen closet and I began sleeping on the mattress of the sofa bed in the lounge room.

The first month was devastating. Every night I felt the absence of the man I had slept with for 17 years, knowing that, unlike the short breaks we had experienced before, this separation was for at least four years while Grace and Gabe finished their secondary schooling.

Every Friday afternoon Nicola and I would pack up clothes for the weekend and drive down to Braidwood and return, sad and bad tempered, on Sunday night. On more than one occasion in that first month, Nicola and/or I would be in tears by the time we arrived at the gate and stay that way for the first half of the seventy minute drive back to Canberra.

It was extraordinary, they were extraordinary; I would leave three teenagers in a house in Canberra for the weekend and return to find, at worst, the washing up not done, and somehow I would still find a reason to be critical. I could sense it but felt powerless to change my pattern. I'm sorry kids, you were/are, all three, extraordinary teenagers.

Even though I felt more appreciative of my relationship with Matthew than ever, I could feel an aspect of my life slipping through my fingers but couldn't identify what it was and what I could do about it. As I look back now it was the illusion of partnership that was fading. Our lives were becoming increasingly separate and there was something about my increasing empowerment that I was enjoying.

Eventually we settled into our new routine and the house took shape. We landed next door to the neighbours from heaven and Nicola spent every moment she could with the three children and a friendship began between our families that continues today.

Gabe and Grace both hit the ground running and blossomed almost immediately. They had been yearning for bigger, broader, and more cosmopolitan and every time they came home bubbling about a new opportunity or friend, I felt both grateful we were able to give them this opportunity and vindicated in our decision to migrate to the city.

I had intended to spend the first couple of months settling in to our new life and writing this book but the cost of living in one of the most expensive cities in Australia was scary and the new feeling of responsibility for my brood, combined to propel me into job-hunting. I found myself a job at a nearby school for distance education, designing maths courses for an internet delivery platform.

Once again I felt like I had landed. I have worked with nice people and have even made friends in the workplace but I have never worked in such a supportive and friendly environment as I found in this distance education centre, particularly in the maths department where I came to be based. More than an income, over the next nine months this job and these people became my stability in an increasingly shifting world.

Life was still tight but we managed – another adventure we approached together.

I set up a place for myself in the corner of the lounge-room that included a desk and a place to practice meditation and yoga. Eventually I got sick of unfolding and refolding the sofa-bed and began sleeping on my yoga mat in this corner.

I would practice last thing before bed and roll out my mat and lie down to sleep, then it was the first thing I did on waking. Nicola would often snuggle up with me on the floor and sometimes we would bring her mattress out for her comfort, but mostly it was the floor and my mat.

It sounds ridiculous but I enjoyed the minimalism, of things and privacy.

Every night after chanting Nicola to sleep, I would absorb myself in writing and then practice; writing for Dru, writing my homework for the yoga course, writing emails, journaling and the beginnings of writing this book.

I think one of the worst things about being a single parent is that I have to both clean the toilet *and* put the garbage out.

It was exhausting, it was demanding but for the first time in my life I began to feel competent. There wasn't another adult to pick up for me when the fatigue of MS washed over me and so I had to use my practice to maintain my function, further embedding it in my life.

Somehow I was starting to feel very grown-up in my new life.

You Belong Because You Exist; You Belong Because You Breathe

MARCH 2009

Towards the end of our first couple of months in Canberra, I had module 7 of the yoga course and module 3 of the meditation within weeks of each other, and my practice shifted into another gear.

The meditation module focussed on the Manomaya kosha, the layer of our being concerned with our motivations in life. We learnt how to focus and amplify our motivation to manifest our goals.

We discovered we couldn't go beyond our own psychic limits and how to identify getting close. We also learned we could expand our limit by regular practice; Andrew called it increasing our fuse rating. I figured the amount of practice I was doing was bound to be increasing my fuse rating and resolved to embrace even the smallest practice as valuable; the same concept as packing, every little bit helps.

Meditation at this level enabled a life I couldn't have imagined even a few months ago. Every day I was still feeling the symptoms of MS but being more productive than I had been for years, and whenever I felt that familiar wave of panic wash over me I would simply breathe myself back into centre and the wave would recede.

I agreed to take a friend's yoga class for the next two terms while she was overseas and, despite the undermining self-doubt, was excited at the prospect of being a yoga teacher again. It always feels so natural for me to be teaching yoga.

The two courses seemed to feed into each other and the friendships formed in both were being consolidated and deepened – for the first time in my life I was feeling like I belonged in life.

I had always said to my children when they were feeling sad or lonely that they belonged because they existed, they belonged because they breathed; even if their place was to sit on the outside that was still *their* place. I knew it to be true but I had never felt it myself, until now.

But even this calm was about to change…

The Storm

APRIL 2009

In April I started to bleed. At first it was just a two-week-long period; annoying, a little draining but not terribly alarming. However, two weeks turned into three, then into four and started to become painful. My next period was due and I hadn't stopped from the previous one.

Then my period hit; intensely painful haemorrhaging that stopped me in my tracks. When the pain came there was nothing else I could do but bend over, sit in the centre and wait for it to pass.

An ultrasound revealed slightly abnormal ovaries but nothing too sinister.

The bleeding didn't stop and was starting to take its toll on both the MS and my iron levels. The vitality I had experienced in the first part of the year was being eroded and I started to feel like an embodied ghost; functioning but ethereal.

I was referred to a specialist and it was agreed to schedule surgery for June to see if we could find out what was the cause of this bleeding. I knew there was a risk of an MS reaction to the general anaesthetic but I also felt obliged to find out if there any structural issue that needed to be sorted.

It seemed the most likely date for the surgery would be June. June was yoga teacher training assessment, not to mention Nicola's birthday – bugger!

I continued to work, teach yoga, go to the Creek each weekend, write and parent but my wellbeing was slipping. At times it seemed like the only thing keeping me on my feet was my practice, which exacerbated my feeling of being ethereal, almost floating through each day on the energy created by meditation.

A Dru nurturing day ended with pain so intense I couldn't speak and an MS moment so potent I couldn't walk or control my muscle spasms. I felt so self-conscious being the person who yoga-ed out of a wheelchair only to be spasming so conspicuously and not even being able to use sticks in the middle of others' calm and wellbeing.

It is difficult to explain the psychology of recovery, particularly for someone who has become an example of healing, and I am sure it is different for everyone so I will speak about my own experiences.

When I made my initial recovery, from the wheelchair to my legs, it was an accidental side effect of my search for peace and I was present to the exciting unfolding of function. It was a childlike discovery of the possibilities.

As it continued and it became clear that my recovery wasn't going to disappear, I started to identify with physical function again and became attached to a certain physical prowess; even to the recovery itself.

It felt quite confusing because on the one hand I felt like I was just doing what I was told and so I thought it was perfectly ordinary.

My teachers had told me I could visualise and so I visualised; Andrew gave me practices at each mentoring session we shared and I did them; and I did the practices at the yoga and meditation modules and then at home.

Trish and Andrew both advocated daily practice and I practiced every day; they advocated reading the Gita and I read the Gita; they advocated giving and gratitude and love, and I did my best. Mentoring with Trish unveiled new levels of understanding and/or new teachings.

Every time I emailed Andrew with an exciting development in my practice he would say 'have fun, it gets better', or something similar. I still felt like I was moving through layers of madness and so I still wasn't satisfied.

I still felt ordinary.

Yet on the other hand, people were saying it was amazing, I was amazing, they told their students about me, my carers were amazed and I started to grow an identity as the person who yoga-ed her way out a wheelchair. As with all identities of the ego it had to be maintained and yoga became a tool of my ego. The ego is such a tricky thing.

So I was ordinary and I was just using the tools and wisdom that had been passed on to me through my teachers and their teachers etc and had a long way to go, yet needed to maintain the ego identity of recovery to which I had become attached.

I still felt MS symptoms every day (still do), but they were the more subtle symptoms and most people didn't notice, and so there was this sense I had cured MS; some people, including my family would even forget that I had it (or perhaps, in the case of my family, that was wishful thinking).

The fluctuating days were easy to mask, not in a deliberate attempt to deceive but to avoid the worried glances, and words of sympathy and advice that came when I slipped. And I so wanted to be undefeatable.

I had forgotten the two most important lessons of my recovery: walking to the beat of my own heart; and that 'surrendering to what is' is the only path to being undefeatable.

My body wasn't allowing for any possibility of masking during the last session of the nurturing day, the most obvious symptoms of mobility loss and whole body spasms left no room for delusion. My brain again felt like fireworks were going off inside.

I was propped up in an armchair to listen to Andrew's final talk, with friends massaging hands and feet and bringing me tea. It was difficult to hold a cup or cutlery so a close friend helped me to eat and drink.

There was an aspect of this that was beautiful and loving and supportive and I felt deeply grateful but there was also an aspect of me that was crumbling, humiliated. When I told my husband, he said "Oh, you would have hated that". He was right; there was an aspect of me that did hate that.

Trish made me a bed in the lounge room and I sat with the flame before bed and again in the morning when I woke, with the focus on calming the pain, soothing my brain, and deeply relaxing my body and mind.

It worked. In the morning I got up and drove down to the Creek to pick up Nicola. There was a hangover and I was still in pain but the intensity had passed, and so had my illusions.

It was now only weeks until my assessment. I had done no preparation and was still bleeding, and I still didn't know when the surgery would be. I discussed the possibilities with Andrew and he once again left the decision in my hands.

This was possibly the most meaningful assessment of my learning life and I really wanted to get it right. Yes, I could use a demonstrator; yes, I could defer, but the ego-identity to which I had become attached wanted to do it myself with the rest of my group. This time I was trying to prove something; prove that I could do it.

Then something happened that showed me I could do my assessment and it wasn't about ego or proving anything. It happened the afternoon of my yoga class.

I was exhausted, still bleeding, feeling MS symptoms and negotiating the registration of our van.

It took longer than I thought it would and cost double what I had thought it was going to, so I had to use the last of my savings to pay for it. I was now broke, again.

I stood on the side of the road in the wind and rain, waiting for the car which was going to be another hour, after which I had to go home, cook dinner, then go out again to teach yoga.

I was empty and I had nothing left to give. And I started to cry. How was I going to teach my class? I couldn't even move out of the rain, let alone teach yoga.

I looked up to the unforgiving sky and, for the second time in my life, I asked for help. I didn't know who I was asking or what I expected but I had nothing left and I needed help.

A short time after, I noticed a cafe I hadn't seen before. I wandered over, ordered a chai latte and found a corner in which to rest. Once upon a time, not that long ago I would have been disdainful of the homeliness of the cafe and its owner but on this day nurturing was exactly what I needed; it was almost as if someone had reached into my emotional state, seen what I needed and provided it in the form of this home away from home, complete with mother-figure-away-from-mother.

I sat and allowed myself to be soothed by the warmth. As soon as I had noticed the cafe while standing in the rain, a spacious calm had settled over my mind, so over the next hour I sat in the warmth and let that calm soak into my bones.

With my car now ready for registration, I returned home to cook dinner and left again to teach my class. I still didn't know how I was going to teach an hour and a half yoga class but I knew I had to do it. The same spacious calm filled my awareness again and I felt the need to trust.

As soon as the students began to arrive my heart opened to them and the idea of teaching the class. I still didn't know how or what I was going to teach but once again I closed my eyes, asked for help and trusted.

Fortunately I had a routine that started every class; welcome, sternum circling and do-in. Out of that practice came the next activation and out of that came the next. That was how the class proceeded, each movement giving birth to the next so the class flowed with grace like an extended Dru sequence.

I felt such love and gratitude as the yoga came through me, not from me. It wasn't the most dynamic yoga class but it was gentle and deeply moving, while retaining the physicality innate in performing yoga asanas and sequences. It was a beautiful class to teach and hopefully a beautiful class to receive.

Now I knew I could do my assessment, regardless of physical state or state of preparedness. I could trust that I could ask for help and yoga would flow through me.

I don't really have the language to adequately describe this experience other than to describe what I felt, as I have done, but the feeling of being supported by a presence beyond the material realm was tangible. The love and gratitude I felt wasn't to someone or something it was just the feeling of love and gratitude.

In the week before the assessment module arrived I felt calm, despite being very unprepared in the typical sense of practice and study and notes, but I knew the sequence and asana intimately and had gone through them in my mind. I had stopped bleeding and decided to demonstrate myself; I didn't really have time to prepare with a demonstrator.

Even still, I woke on the morning of the actual assessment and realised I hadn't really done enough technical preparation (contra-indications, alignment points, timing etc), and it was too late to cram now. I also realised I already was a yoga teacher and would eventually pass if I didn't pass today. I would be a qualified Dru teacher, sooner later and in that knowledge I let go of the pass/fail thing, deciding instead to offer my peers something that was me; I wanted to give them something of myself.

At that moment the mood around my assessment shifted and spacious calm descended. I came home at lunch to work out my activations and promptly fell over during one of them. Grace, who was having a mental health day, burst into laughter and we both laughed, before deciding to omit that one from my *class*.

I was the last to teach and the groups was exhausted and flatter than a collective pancake after yoga-ing, teaching and supporting all day; so through the activation I slowly built up the energy until we were all laughing and happily yoga-ing again.

After a brief pause I took them through the sitting spinal twist, inviting my peers to feel the release at each vertebra as we twisted the spine and felt the opening of our hearts.

My assessment sequence was Seat of Compassion sequence. I began by sharing three stories of compassion (see *The three stories of compassion p.305)* I had recently experienced and invited my *students* to perform the sequence with the intention of compassion. It was lovely to bring my life into yoga and yoga into life.

There was a sense of reverence and stillness in the room that was beyond the physical movements of the sequence.

I was now running over time, so I relaxed the physical body in pairs (both legs, both arms) so I could give them some time in stillness. I had planned to chant the ancient mantra of light, too, and even if I could only do it once, I still wanted to do the chant. I wanted to offer my peers the opportunity of filling their bodies with light in a state of relaxation, even though I wasn't sure if it would compromise my pass or fail.

Finally it was done and I felt so happy. I felt like I had failed on technicalities but had succeeded in being myself, and giving my peers something of me and my practice. In all my life I had never felt so confidant in giving my essence ... and the technicalities would come with practice.

As my peers packed up their mats and joined the other group and the teachers I spent a few moments in deep gratitude for the gift I had been given and the gift I gave; passing or failing seemed insignificant.

The rest of the module went so smoothly. I have

never experienced the bonding and the camaraderie I felt during those four days. MS was present after my assessment, and doctor appointments and Nicola's birthday took me away from the module, but the spirit of deep friendship and love we gave each other was embedded in my soul.

Oh, and I passed.

Three Stories of Compassion

The Christian, the Hare Krishnas and the Muslim
Compassion comes in many forms, in the guise of all religions
and secular movements; ultimately, the decision to express
compassion in our lives rests with the individual.

The Christian

There is a road in Canberra called Hindmarsh Drive that
stretches from Fyshwick in the east all the way across the
south of Canberra to Weston in the west. And there is a point
on that road, driving west when you round a bend at the
top of hill and the panorama of south Canberra opens up in
front of you. The city is edged with the Brindabellas and the
sky is huge, and at sunset the ever-changing canvas of pink
and orange and purple, tinged with blue, is breathtaking. I
have loved this spectacular view ever since I began driving to
Canberra.

It was at this point in the road one day, on the way from

work to a mentoring session with Trish, that I began to feel the slight lean and hear the telltale noises of a flat tyre. I pulled over on to verge and investigated. Yep, a flat on the front left. Bugger! I had never changed a tyre before and I was driving our 4-wheel-drive van.

The first thing I did was call Matthew. What do I do? His first advice was to stand by the car and look helpless – someone would stop and help. No! I wanted to at least try and do it myself.

So there I was on the side of the road in Canberra in late autumn with the panorama of sunset spreading across the sky, getting wheel changing instructions over my mobile. I found the spare and the jack, and then tried to loosen the nuts on the wheel.

They were so tight I couldn't make them budge. Then with sheer determination and the extra leverage of standing on the tool, the first nut began to move; just a micro move-ment but it was definitely a movement. Then one by one all the nuts moved, enough to know I could actually get the wheel off.

Next was getting the car jacked up. The car was facing down hill so I needed wedges for wheels. Done. Then finding the point for the jack – not so easy. The height of the jack didn't seem to match the height of the van.

At this point a car pulled up and a young man offered to help. I had not given up, had proved to myself I was not incompetent and I could now accept help and I did. It was a difficult task to get the van jacked up but he continued, despite being late for a meeting.

As it came to pass, the man who had come to my aide

was a born again Christian, and as he was changing the wheel on my car he was also hoping to save my soul. He didn't stop to save my soul but he genuinely wanted to bring God into my life.

He didn't stop changing my wheel when I didn't renounce yoga; he just genuinely wanted what he thought was the best for me. I was deeply touched by his efforts with my wheel and his attempts for my spirit as I watched the beautiful panorama of sunset over Canberra evolve before me.

The Hare Krishnas

A chance meeting at a lovely cafe on the South Coast of NSW led to a friendship with a Hare Krishna couple; he was so gentle and full of peace and his wife so full of exhuberance. A short time later they came to my house in Canberra with their van full of utensils to cook dinner for my family and a few friends.

They cooked, served and cleaned up. We ate beautiful food, chanted a little and listened to a satsang (a discussion about spirituality and the Gita). I guess they were selling books and maybe recruiting but it was a generous offering, and a beautiful way to share something that was so precious to their lives.

The next time they came to Canberra they called again. This time I was feeling the effects of the bleeding and the worsening MS, so I couldn't offer to host a dinner for my friends. Not a problem, they would cook dinner for my family, for me.

Once again, they arrived with their van full of utensils and food, and cooked a beautiful meal for my family and myself, and cleaned up as well. This time there were no books or satsang, it was just pure open-hearted generosity for someone they hardly knew, and I accepted with the love with which it was offered.

The Muslim

I think sometimes in our society we have a view of Islam as a religion of extremists due to the international media coverage of the Middle East conflict and Islamic terrorism. Yet in focussing on the fundamentalist expression of Islam we forget about the millions of Muslims living peacefully in the West and the East.

Our minds have been filled with images by an insatiable media machine, but an incident in early June reminded me of the fallacy of such generalisations. A Muslim, a quiet and gentle man, was being harassed by someone who was making accusations about Islam based on their misunderstanding of Islamic theology.

This man gently and peacefully defended his religion. He returned none of the aggression he was receiving but patiently explained where these misunderstandings arise and the truth of the Koran. He had read the Koran first in English then in Arabic to understand it more deeply.

It was fascinating listening to him talk about the Koran: as transforming as listening to anyone talking about their love of spirit in such a peaceful, dignified way. I realised how little I knew about Islam and the Koran, and he offered to teach me.

There was nothing to be gained by him in this offer but freely sharing his love of spirit and his spirituality; something as precious as his family.

To bear witness to his dignity under fire was truly inspirational and opened my heart to the need to be generous of spirit to the spirit in everyone.

Five Weeks Until Surgery

JUNE – AUGUST 2009

After assessment I felt a huge relief. A burden had been lifted from my shoulders but there was also a sense of validation I had not expected.

I had been teaching for almost a year but the class I taught after the assessment felt different; somehow passing my assessment had given licence to be standing in front of a group of people as a yoga teacher. There was a confidence and entitlement in my teaching that hadn't been there, even the week before.

There was now about five weeks until my surgery and there were tasks I needed to finish. I was again in pregnant-woman-about-to-drop mode. There was writing to be done for Dru, a course to finish at work, work to be done at home as well as my own writing.

I think I became obsessed with being super teacher/cripple/mother/Drubee and sacrificed everything to finish; everything except my practice, which was what kept me functioning. Even so, it was a brittle, thin layer of functioning that could have served as a danger sign; a flashing warning of impending doom.

Nonetheless, a calm and joy was descending upon me the closer it came to the date of my surgery. I knew there was a danger of another exacerbation and felt unsure as to what the result of that would be, and what the result of the surgery itself would be, yet I felt peaceful.

Two nights before the surgery I put Nicola to sleep and I went over to the Dru office to help finalise a mail out. One of the core team and I were sitting in a room, she working on her computer and me packing envelopes, when she stopped and laughed.

I looked at her quizzically and she said she had looked over to me while I was working and saw a beaming smile on my face as I stuffed envelopes with leaflets. That was just how I felt.

The following night at midnight I finally finished all my tasks. All the writing, all the housework and course work was done. Now I could relax and focus on surrender.

Surrender is golden

I awoke from the surgery and noticed I couldn't swallow. The nurse brought ice or ice water and I couldn't swallow. Then I noticed I couldn't lift my head. OK, not that unusual after surgery, I suppose; maybe still groggy from the anaesthetic. After a little negotiation with admissions, I was transferred to a ward and more tests.

It was discovered I couldn't take weight on my arms or legs, or sense the fullness of my bladder. My blood pressure and heart rate were dangerously low, my breathing rate was also compromised and there was no evidence of a gag reflex.

"Nil by mouth", IV, catheter and oxygen mask.

Again there was that sense of contained panic in the people around me. Yet within the hustle and bustle, I felt a deep sense of calm. This was what I had felt before; profound surrender.

All morning I had prepared with meditation and relaxation, preparing to accept whatever the outcome of the surgery, regarding both MS and my reproductive system. When I woke up with dysfunction I surrendered, and what followed was golden; peaceful relaxation to what was.

The next day breakfast came, neither gluten-free nor easy to swallow; it was funny. Then a very caring nursing sister decided I needed a shower and ordered the shower hoist. Thankfully the hoist came with a very capable staff member, because the sister hadn't realised I had so little muscle tone.

My neck flopped, my arms flopped and my legs flopped; catheter tubes and bag, IV tube and bag; I was hanging in mid-air with hospital gown gracefully parting at the rear, while everything was sorted.

Then we left on my elastic stockings in the shower and they were soaked; I dropped the shower head and saturated the bathroom; and each time I was left on the shower chair I slid to one side or the other. It was a comedy of errors and all I could do was laugh.

As I look back at that time, even I am surprised by how relaxed and patient I was; I just felt so appreciative that these people of our health system were going to such effort to give me a shower.

Each day my condition improved, and I returned home on Monday having spent three days in hospital for a day surgery procedure. A small quantity of endometriosis tissue was removed and all else was good, and while my mobility was still compromised, all tubes were removed. Now it was just a matter of time.

The surrender I felt during these few days was golden. The acceptance of my circumstances generated pure joy and this joy was just as valid as joy derived from more desirable circumstances.

Recovery

After a quick visit to my home in Canberra, Matthew took Nicola and me back to Majors Creek. There was a sense of comfort in returning to Braidwood in a wheelchair; I had been here before, I knew what this was like and the surrender was still golden. Yet it was also confronting; an element of defeat invaded my surrender.

I had forgotten how uncomfortable wheelchairs are, how instantly people suddenly know what is best for you, how far you should try to recover, and how much you should relax. It was almost like the previous 18 months had been negated in people's minds by the effects of the general anaesthetic. I thought I had demonstrated my ability to assess and choreograph my own recovery but it seems being in a wheelchair is not only a symbol of immobility but also incompetence.

Intellectually I understood that concern for my wellbeing was motivating the advice but emotionally I wanted to shout and scream and rebel; once again I felt throttled in my relationships with people.

Unlike the time after the previous surgery when I was busy visualising sequences and postures, my overwhelming instinct this time was to be still and listen; to notice the thoughts that were coming up. My only practice was meditation and relaxation. With Andrew's guidance, via email and text, I focussed on acceptance of self.

I got out of my chair each day to walk as far as I could with my sticks but the compulsion to walk had diminished. I noticed the distance increasing with a detached eye; 1 metre, 2 metres etc but I had a deep knowing that it would happen in its own time... or not.

These moments of surrender were golden.

Yet still I struggled with my pride and my return to dependence; I had been so functional and independent and here I was again, at times needing my six-year-old to push my wheelchair because there was no strength in either arms or legs.

And wheelchairs are uncomfortable! The chair I was in was the right size but I had forgotten the valuable techniques of cushioning and supporting my body in sitting. By the third or fourth day I could feel my posture deteriorating and the distant yet familiar pain in my diaphragm, back and neck from the collapse in the front of my body, as well as constriction of my breath.

Instinctively, I started to raise the base of my sternum (the very base of my breastbone), and felt my chest open, shoulder blades come closer together and my crown rise. At the same the spot behind my shoulder blades that I had wanted to scratch (like it was irritable) was being stimulated and soothed, creating a release of energy from the heart.

The temporary relief was astonishing so I started to explore techniques for a deeper opening.

The arm movements from EBR 1 came into mind (see **Wheelchair yoga** p.317). Again, the relief was instant. Fatigue was a serious symptom again so I rediscovered the value of small bits of practice often.

Instantly my breathing was relieved and the pain throughout my body was eased.

After a week at Majors Creek, I returned home to Canberra. My condition had improved but I was still very tired, and while I could walk short distances around the house, I tired easily and needed the wheelchair for any movement outside the house; even getting in and out of the car was difficult.

Matthew had been planning a return trip to the UK to see his family for some time. The flights had been booked and paid for months before. The original departure date was three days after my surgery. After I woke with the relapse, he decided to delay his departure for a week so he could look after me in the acute phase of my recovery. So the day after we returned to Canberra, Matthew left Australia.

Two lovely friends came with food and I was

able to get funding for post-hospital recovery for the following eight weeks. Once again we survived and once again I recovered.

Within weeks I resumed teaching yoga, my part-time job and being a single parent, but as the more obvious symptom of extreme fatigue and mobility receded, the more subtle symptoms of MS became more noticeable.

Balance, dexterity, stamina, hearing, eyesight and sensation were all compromised; I missed the vitality I had experienced before I had started bleeding for 12 weeks. My GP decided it was time to revisit a neurologist.

Wheelchair yoga

The quick solution for the symptoms of sitting a lot is to lift the sternum vertically, putting a slight pressure behind the heart.

Side bends
- *Place your left hand in front of your navel, palm up. Elongate your spine and raise your right arm sideways and overhead. Your palm faces down as though you are holding a large beach ball between your hands. Lift and stretch from the right elbow.*
- *Bend over to the left, stretching from the right hip through to your shoulder and into your right hand.*
- *Engage your core stability muscles, breathe*

---

in and straighten up, lifting from the right elbow. Your arms reverse positions symmetrically as you rise up, as if you are rolling the beach ball between your hands.

- *Repeat two more times to each side.*

Arm Rotations

- *With your arms a little distance away from your sides, rotate them forwards. The movement flows from the shoulders, into the elbows and wrists.*
- *Rotate your arms backwards, beginning the movement from the shoulders. Feel your chest opening.*
- *Continue the rotations, gradually raising your arms to shoulder height.*
- *Rotate your arms in alternate directions so that one arm rolls forwards at the same time as the other one rolls backwards. Your head turns in the direction of the upturned hand.*
- *Extend your arms on the out-breath, release and twist on the in-breath and then reverse.*
- *Lower your arms to your side.*
- *Shoulder circling*
- *Place your fingertips on your shoulders with your elbows in front.*
- *Keeping your fingers on your shoulders, draw your elbows up and above your head. Raise your head slightly as you lengthen your upper spine. Keep your shoulders and neck relaxed throughout.*

- *Take your elbows back and out to the sides as you lower them as though drawing circles with your elbows. Complete the circular movement, raising the elbows in front, and repeat the movements.*
- *Repeat two more times.*
- *Reverse the movements, breathing in as you raise your elbows behind you and out as you lower them in front.*
- *Repeat two more times, then lower your arms to your sides.*

  The quick fix is to breathe up through the spine, lift the breastbone and gently roll the shoulders but a quick warning: once you start, it feels so good you will want to do all three stretches, so be prepared.

Separation

Meanwhile another crisis was looming in my life. While Matthew was overseas it became apparent the physical separation that had begun in January was being completed, emotionally. Six years of crises, including MS, had taken its toll and we were done. The emotional pain was excruciating.

I have since heard that when one partner undergoes a healing journey of some significance (eg chronic or terminal illness), the personal growth required is so great that it often means the other partner is 'left behind'. Many relationships do not survive this disparity in personal development.

I wonder if this is part of what happened to us?

Regardless, it is not possible to describe 17½ years of relationship and its breakdown in the space I want to give it here, so I won't. Suffice it to say I was emotionally exhausted. The wave of unsaid and unfelt emotions felt like being hit in the back with semi-trailer or a freight train.

In the weeks that followed I felt like I was on an emotional roller coaster. I really wanted to be compassionate and wise but waves of anger overwhelmed me. My practice brought me out but each time it happened I felt devastated; like I was failing. Finally I pleaded to be released from this angst.

Losing My Mind

We all have something about ourselves we value. Even those of us stuck in the illusion of self-hatred (and this has been me for most of my life) have something in our personality that we love; we have pride, even hubris, about this quality. This is the aspect of us that gives us a status or specialness in the world; that sets us apart from everyone else.

You may be able to recognise it by thinking of the quality that enables you to feel some superiority over others and when it is threatened by meeting someone you perceive may be superior to you in this aspect, you instantly feel defensive and perhaps even resentful and aggressive toward that person. That's it; that's the quality you value about yourself above all others in your personality.

For me that quality is my mind — I love my mind. I love the way it thinks, I love the way it is so eclectic.

I love that it is capable of distilling the essence out of the issue and working with the essence. I love that it is so anarchic in its refusal to follow other people's rules just because they exist. I love its analytical ability. And I really love that its intellectual capability to learn has meant I have never had to study very much to achieve academic progress.

And yes, I have felt certain smugness that my mind has put me in an elite group of the population; as the gifted and talented speak goes, the top 5-10% of the population in terms of intellectual potential. And yes, this smugness has also given me the opportunity to feel both superiority and its mirror twin, inferiority, because no matter how good you are at something, there will always be someone else who is better.

One thing we can all be certain of is that when the ego wages war on 'other', it also wages war on the self. When we feel justified in feeling superior to others because in some way we are 'better', we will automatically feel 'less' when we meet someone who threatens our superiority. And the more we are attached to our feeling of superiority, the deeper the perceived inferiority cuts.

It is not that I have thought I am the most intelligent person in the world and certainly not the highest academic achiever (I have worn out the seat of my pants, flying on it in that respect) but I love to think; think out of the square, left of centre, out of the box and whatever other euphemism there exists for thinking independently and analytically. I am the personification of the pink hippo facing in the opposite direction. And, well, secretly, I love it … no, I don't just love, I pride myself on it.

Can you see the danger?

So, over my short dance with MS, I have let go of the need for mobility, flexibility and strength, in fact any form of physical prowess; I have surrendered to loss of bladder control, career permanence, sense perception, perfect speech and vision and stamina. Age was taking care of vanity, and illness and babies were dealing with our cultural obsession of being slim and having flat bits everywhere.

I have watched other sufferers of chronic illness rise above their illness by becoming well or advocates or both, even other people with MS becoming yoga teachers before me – outrageous! The world is full of inspiring people, so little room for ego in my reality, you would think.

Aaah, not so, when the effluent hits the fan on all other fronts, I can always retreat to my beautiful, independent mind. Can you see how in love with my mind I was and hence how vulnerable I was?

I believed I could learn anything and to some degree I had proved myself right. Through my life I have become apprentice in many trades and master of none. I have learned many skills across many fields at a basic level and some at more than a basic level just because I believed there was nothing my mind couldn't learn.

So what happens to a mind that loves to think but

is confused, forgetful and can't concentrate; that lives in a perpetual fog not even able to deal with the basics of personal management like filling out forms or writing consent notes; a maths tutor who sometimes has to pause to count?

First step, denial!

Next step, find something else to learn where you don't need to analyse.

For me that was Dru Yoga and Meditation – the ego is such a tricky thing.

When I started the Dru Yoga Teacher Training, it was to learn to live and love in peace, to learn to teach yoga to other people with chronic illness and disability… and because I didn't think I would be able to teach maths for very long.

Initially it was great; learning the postures and sequences seemed to come naturally and my concentration improved markedly, so soon my mind was feeling happily superior once again. But then the anatomy and the Sanskrit and contra-indications and the benefits and, and, and…

Well, clearly the anatomy wasn't that important and neither was the Sanskrit (completely ignoring the fact that sometimes I forgot the English names) so that was OK. And the contra-indications I learned by learning the essence of why it wasn't good to do certain groups of postures with certain conditions. It kind of became common sense after a while. Then the benefits were also common sense to some degree and I am still learning every time I go to help at a teaching module.

I could ignore those times when my brain seemed to stop due to tiredness because that was…well…due to tiredness; mind/ego happy again.

And then another relapse; initially the focus was again on the loss of mobility and stamina because they are the gross symptoms that people notice. Surrender to immobility is relatively easy but the loss of my hands is more difficult. Nonetheless, surrender is golden and my recovery continued.

It was only after a few weeks when the more obvious symptoms were dissipating that the more subtle symptoms became more apparent. Visual disturbances, concentration lapses (the lapse was becoming more common than the concentration), hearing impairment, but still I acknowledge them only in the very secret part of my mind.

Even my beloved meditation and yoga practice was becoming more difficult to sustain. My mind couldn't sustain stillness or visualisation for very long at a time so I found myself practicing in tiny bits again. While I know this is perhaps a better practice for life, my mind wanted the long sits and the ability to visualise a class, and I felt restless and dissatisfied.

A visit to a new neurologist in Sydney and I was forced to see the reality of MS and cognitive dysfunction.

"The majority of untreated MS sufferers have to leave work within five years of diagnosis, not because of mobility issues but because of the effect on the mind." Bang! I felt like I had just been hit over the head with a 4x2 – ouch!

I was reeling with panic and fear. I realised losing my mind, my ability to think (and suffering clinical depression again – one of the side affects of one class of MS drugs), was my greatest fear ... and this fear was my greatest enemy in making coherent decisions.

I had a month to have another MRI scan and a visual field test... a month's grace.

Once again I was saved by my yoga practice and the intention to release the hold ego has over most of us through this life.

The following words were written a couple of days after the visit with the neurologist.

Transforming fear

There is so much fear in the world, so much pain, so much anger. Imagine what life would be like if we could walk away from our fear; imagine if we could walk away from our pain and anger, stop blaming the people we meet and the circumstances we experience. What would that be like?

Last night a miracle occurred for me. Last night I found out what it would be like and it is freedom. Last night I taught a Dru yoga class.

There seem so many decisions to make and they all carry some, if not all of the above mentioned elements, and every time I put my head above water to gasp for air the undertow of emotion pulls me back down under. How can I make clear decisions about my future when my present seems so clouded by whirling emotions; like trying to see clearly through pea-soup fog?

I am able to rescue myself for intermittent periods with my spiritual practice and/or teaching Dru. I discover the strength of my faith and the strength it gives me and I discover using my pain to help others is incredibly powerful, for them and for me … but I want to turn my face toward the Sun and stay there.

The context of this feeling is the resumption of ongoing bleeding (about four weeks so far) and a new diagnosis of premenopause with no ovulation or progesterone production. The conventional medical solution is a five year slow release progesterone IUD; one naturopath suggested progesterone ointment, and another prescribed remedies to encourage the pituitary to behave, with both wanting to support my deplet- ed system to regenerate.

This is combined with the final dissolution of my rela- tionship with my husband. Many others thought it inevitable but I didn't until afterwards. Seventeen years of unexpressed pain and recriminations came flooding to the surface. I felt overwhelmed by waves of grief and anger. I so wanted to want the best for him but couldn't. I felt like I was failing; failing myself, my spiritual path, the people who had had faith in me and all the people I might have helped if I had managed to get this right.

Yet all the while there existed a presence, a knowing, a solidity underneath the emotion. Each time my head rose for air, a recognition that I was still here emerged.

The final blow came with the uncompromising honesty from the neurologist. I think professionals in the world of MS management soften the reality in order to prevent the onset of depression and hopelessness. But when a highly qualified experienced medical specialist tells you that most MS patients are not working within five years of diagnosis, not due to mobility issues but cognitive dysfunction, it is shocking.

Drug therapy, immediately – self-injected interferon (immunosuppressant). The deterioration incurred by not taking the therapy will never be caught up, even if I start the therapy down the track.

I had avoided this discussion by not having a definite diagnosis but there was no doubt in the mind of this doctor. There was a reprieve – a spinal and brain MRI and a visual evoked response test followed by an appointment to discuss the results. At least I had a month.

I have to negotiate a property settlement, decide on living arrangements for my family and make major decisions about my health on two fronts.

Once again, my life has thrown itself up and everything seems to be negotiable.

Amidst absent friends and the ever shifting sands of life, the only things I trust are my love for my children, my relationship with my spirit, my Dru practice/teaching and the Gita.

I knew fear and pain were obstructing my view of the world and knew I would have to get past them to make clear decisions … but how?

Then last night, after a day of communicating with my husband, I was cleaning my teeth in preparation for teaching my yoga class and felt a deep yearning to be free of angst about the past.

There is a rune that talks about standing on the edge of a cliff with your past behind you and your future in front, then stepping off. This was the image in my mind with a hand *gently pushing me, as I was spitting out my toothpaste.*

Who would have thunk it? Such a deep spiritual request made while undertaking such a mundane activity as cleaning my teeth. It goes to show that a life is made up of small moments and one must be paying attention to all of them; that retreats and workshops and euphoric meditations are no replacements for practice and awareness in one's everyday life.

So I taught my yoga class: activation, EBR3 and Seat of Compassion sequence and a therapy, followed by a relaxation.

EBR3, for me, is about opening the heart, setting a goal from your heart and sending energy after that goal. While I teach, the yoga seems to come through me so I feel the transformative effects of the practices as my students do.

The image of the cliff-top came into my mind when it came time to set the goal and the concept of leaving the angst behind articulated by stepping off the cliff. The energy propelled by the last movement in EBR 3 was the hand behind my heart pushing me toward my goal.

Then the Seat of Compassion, a most transformative sequence. I had been teaching the sequence for four weeks, focussing on compassion but this time I talked about transforming fear, but to what?

For me it was trust. So I embraced trust and released fear, then finally extended to all those people suffering similar struggles to myself, and encouraged the class to do the same.

It was extraordinary. I quite literally, felt fear being released. I felt the light come into my eyes.

My students gave each other a beautiful massage therapy

and then I chanted the ancient mantra of light during the relaxation.

Today I have experienced a lightness of being I didn't think was possible. My circumstances haven't changed but the fear and angst surrounding my view of them has. I can think about the issues, clearly.

And the final miracle was the experience of oneness; the actual experience of oneness as reality – no separation. There is now no question of being loved or not; love just is and I am part of it.

There may be times in the future when these emotions return but now I know there is both a deeper reality and various tools to navigate me towards it. And if there are tools of transformation for me, there are tools for others as well.

So I have faced losing my body and now I am facing losing my beautiful mind, and yet I am still here. I have reflected on the times of fog and realised that the moments when I have surrendered to intellectual humility have been the times of greatest expressions of the essence of who I am. There is no need for fear, I will find another way to earn a living other than teaching maths and science, even other than teaching yoga if I have to because I am still here.

I am reminded of two of my favourite quotes.

First from Deepak Chopra:

"I am not my body, I am not my mind; I have a body and I have a mind."

And then, from the Gita:

"Sarva dharman pratyaja,
maam ekam sharanam vraja,
aham tva sarva parpebyo,

moksha yishyami maa suchah."

"Letting go of everything else, with your whole heart, take refuge in Me for I will free you of everything that causes you pain. There is no need for fear or worry."

What a Day

I left home at 7am to drive to Sydney for a test on my optic nerve, and a brain and spinal MRI.

Just over an hour north of Canberra I had an altercation with a double semi-trailer and was bumped off the road onto the grassy verge; the corner of his bull bar collided with the middle of my tailgate. My life went in to slow motion and my mind became clear. Fortunately, the van I was driving was 4wd and I was able to drive it back on to the tar, with no further damage to me or the car.

The truck pulled in to the merging lane in front of me and there was a moment when the world seemed to stop. Again my first reaction was to change my breath and move into a meditative state. I sat in the car and consciously relaxed my body and mind.

When I felt centred I got out of the car and approached the truck; despite the feeling of jelly in my legs and the remnants of the feeling of my bowels going to water in my mind, I felt so calm. The truck driver was on his phone so I waited until he was finished. He was so angry, blamed me and said he was calling the police. I was working on surrender, so I thanked him for calling the police and went back to van.

I walked around to the back of the car and found a deep crease down the centre of the tailgate. The window was smashed and the rear bumper bar was trashed but the car looked drivable.

L-shaped meditation (see *L-shaped meditation* p.339), breathe and surrender. I consciously slowed everything down and concentrated on staying relaxed and feeling the surrender flow through my mind and body. I felt so blessed and grateful for being alive.

I alternated between meditation and scanning through my body for the places where I was holding on to the tension of crisis. Each time I located the crisis I used my out-breath to release the tension. I didn't want to hold on to anything after the need had passed. I called Matthew and the Dru office (fortunately I spoke with one of the senior tutors and her voice alone was enough to bring extra calm).

After what seemed like an eternity the policeman came. He was the nicest man and talked to us both separately before talking to us both. Essentially, he decided not to carry out a formal investigation of the accident. He gave us both his details if either of us decided to pursue the matter further and left the scene.

So, after about an hour of meditating for the highest

good and breathing to release the crisis and panic from my system, the truck driver finally left after putting an arm around my shoulders and wishing me well.

Matthew arrived a little later and we both went back to Goulburn – I needed grounding with food and chai! I had told him I didn't need rescuing and if he was coming to rescue me, to stay in Braidwood but if he genuinely wanted to help then it would be lovely to see him. And it was lovely to see him.

Matthew and I were able to have the most important conversation as I explained the healing I had experienced around my beliefs regarding relationships and he opened a little more about his own process. Our life as a married couple was over but it seemed a friendship was possible and I felt good about that.

I drove down to Braidwood to drop off the van so Matt could oversee the repairs and he drove me back to Canberra.

Gabe had missed the bus to meet his girlfriend at Swing Dance class so I drove him over to O'Connor. On returning at about 6.50, I called the friend who was looking after Nicola to see how she was going and discovered she was sick; a few mouthfuls of veggie casserole and off to get her.

When I arrived she was starting to become feverish and was complaining of a sore tummy, bent over like an old person. This is very unusual for Nicola because she is rarely sick. I was concerned she might have appendicitis so I took her off to Emergency. We arrived at around 7.30pm.

A little while later the admissions nurse measured her temperature at 40° and gave her Panadol. Then around 9.30pm she was still complaining about tummy ache and feverish, so I laid her down on one of the sofas in the waiting room, and massaged and stroked her back, finally resting my hands at the top and base of her spine.

After a while, her temperature decreased, the tummy ache was soothed and she went to sleep. I was sitting on the floor next to her lying down on the sofa where I stayed for the next couple of hours.

Finally around midnight, we were taken into the Emergency ward and she was seen by a doctor. Probably not appendicitis but it can start this way so keep an eye on her. She does have an infection, and swollen lymph nodes in the abdomen may be the cause of the pain. A bottle of Panadol and we were done. We came home; I put her to bed, ate, had some chai and downloaded, in an email, to Andrew and Trish.

"How truly wonderful that spiritual practice can be so practical. How wonderful that I can do this. I am tired but my mind is clear, I don't feel like I am carrying baggage from the day. Although, having said that, I am feeling the effects of a mortality call; one of those 'pulling back the veil of permanence to reveal what is real' moments.

One must be so present, even when the circumstances are not pleasant. Presence and surrender enable beauty to come out of the most unlikely events.

One must take every interaction as an opportunity to surrender, let go of ego and be in that part of one's self that is love. And stop wasting time. And be ready to throw all plans out the window to be present for the people who need me the most."

At 2am I finally went to bed, twenty hours after getting up the previous day. I had survived.

Nicola and I had the next day at home together. Her tummy pain and fever returned, and I did the same thing as I had the night before. Her tummy ache and fever abated, as it did the following day. Of course, had the fever and the pain persisted, I would have returned to the doctor, but fortunately it wasn't necessary.

For someone who was recovering from an MS exacerbation and had the mother of all interesting days, I felt exhausted but strangely calm and functional. Over the following couple of days I was then able to give time at the teacher training module taking place in Canberra that weekend. I felt so blessed to have been able to use my practice to make my life possible, again.

L-shaped Meditation

The L-shaped meditation is a quick and easy meditation you can use to transform your experience of difficult situations in your life, return a sense of control and hence possibly alter the outcome.

- *Focus on the challenging situation as it is, visualising it in front of your heart*
- *Breathe into your heart and out of your crown into the space above your head*
- *Visualise light or an intention in the space*

above your head
- *Breathe it in through your crown, down into your heart*
- *Breathe out from your heart into the situation in front of your heart*
- *Repeat this until the situation in front of your heart changes*
- *You can return to this process as many times as you like until you no longer feel the need*

In the time immediately following the collision with the truck, I worked with the intention of the highest good for all and that was exactly the result.

What Happened Next?

OCTOBER 2009

What unfolded over the following weeks was astonishing, even for me who has been living through a pretty extraordinary journey already. I experienced a grace and serendipity I thought was only the stuff of myths and legends; certainly not in my humble life.

The bleeding was resolved by the naturopathic remedies, and the necessity for the progesterone IUD bypassed (in the context of MRI, this is a good thing). My body began to rebuild itself and I began to feel feminine for the first time in my life (I know this sounds strange, but I have battled with my femininity all my life and during this period I began to really feel like a woman).

I had an incredible day where I was able to maintain equanimity through some very trying circumstances (see, **What a day!**), through my now natural use of my spiritual tools. I think my first words to one my teachers, was, "This stuff actually works. What we teach actually works in real life!"

This was a critical point for me where I actually understood in real terms the power of living in spiritual consciousness. And by that I mean using the tools of spirituality in everyday life to tackle everyday issues.

There is a line in the Rune Book that recommends we live the ordinary life in an extraordinary way, and I think this is what I was and am still doing. About a year into my yoga teacher training, I wrote to one of my teachers, "heaven is a state of mind, not a real estate location", and now I know what I meant.

Regarding MS, I waxed and waned between drugs and no drugs, each time adamant that that was the right decision; I flowed between the extremes. A local support group taught me not to be scared of the side effects; that there is a drug that doesn't have depression as a side effect (I have been depressed and I would rather be in a wheelchair and not be able to think than be chronically depressed).

Then, at some point of clarity I realised each side was clouded by fear and ego: no drugs, I wanted to do it with yoga and meditation, I wanted to be the person to show it could be done and I didn't want depression again; and drugs, I didn't want to lose my ability to think. So, I realised I had to find the space between fear and ego, and slip into it to make my decision.

In my mind, the two sides formed an arch, with a small patch of light between. I stepped into that light with the question in my mind. The answer came clearly and immediately – if the tests show deterioration, take the drugs. The decision was clear and peace returned to my mind. In the days before I went back to the neurologist, I checked in several times to test the clarity of my decision and it didn't waiver. If anything the decision became stronger, more certain.

So when I sat in the neurologist's office and we looked at the scans and discussed my slow visual responses, the decision was clear and easy. Drugs. The prescription was written and I spent an hour being 'educated' about self-injecting.

I was about to move so I decided to wait until after the move, but when I arrived home I realised that I needed to start immediately and put the prescription into the local pharmacy.

Having decided to take the drugs I wanted to embrace the new regime, and create a new ritual that maximised the potential of the drugs and minimised the potential side-effects. I didn't know if it would help in physical terms but it was a perspective thing – if I changed my perspective then my experience of my circumstances would change, and if I welcomed the drugs psychologically then maybe my body would too.

I needed to find a ritual I would do every day at the same time; loved doing every day at the same time. Never having been a person of great routine, the only thing I did every day at the same time was my morning spiritual practice. Every morning I woke, sat at my altar and meditated; and I loved my practice.

What better solution than to incorporate my daily

injections into my morning meditation practice? Each morning I would rise and put the pre-filled syringe on my altar and meditate; and finally, chant and give myself my injection.

I know it sounds very ooby-gooby but it was amazing, I welcomed the injections; the first one was almost euphoric, with only a small swelling afterwards and no other side effects.

Over the following weeks, I felt amazing as the fatigue that had plagued me since the surgery began to lift. I didn't know if it was the drugs or the new intensity of my practice or just coincidence (perhaps placebo) but the difference was clear and undeniable.

The injection itself was relatively painless but the moments after were quite painful as the drug was absorbed into my system. I was determined not to retain any tension around the injection and so practiced relaxation and chanted during the pain; the acute phase took about ten to fifteen minutes to subside and an ache was left for about an hour before subsiding completely.

The swelling at the site of injection was tender for a day or so but there were a number of sites I could inject into, so each site had recovered by the time the cycle returned to it.

In essence, I had accepted this was my life and adjusted to my new regime; and I was beginning to feel alive again.

Maybe I'm Not a Fraud

NOVEMBER 2009

One of the things you might notice when you go to any Dru Australia event, particularly the training courses, is the number of helpers standing around the edges of the room, waiting to bring rescue remedy or water or prepare the morning tea or help with questions about posture or practice or even just a friendly conversation in the break times.

I felt incredibly supported and cared for at my first module when the helpers were introduced from Canberra, Sydney, Brisbane, Melbourne and Albury. I wondered if this was just a one-off for our first module, but every subsequent module for both the yoga and meditation courses was the same; and when I realised all those people were coming as volunteers, the feeling of being nurtured in part of a national network of yogis was even more accentuated.

The thought of these people giving up weekends

and travelling to Canberra to support us through this journey was extraordinary, so when I came close to finishing my teacher training course I wanted to give new students the same feeling of being nurtured and supported in their personal journey and teacher training.

I went to help on a Sydney weekend and it was such an amazing experience to be giving back to the process that had been so therapeutic for me.

Of course, I felt like I didn't know anything and a little like a spare leg but it was wonderful nonetheless. In addition to helping it was another learning experience; an opportunity to learn the postures and techniques again, at a different level. I realised that if I was serious about becoming a yoga teacher this was a very good way of continuing my education while doing something useful.

Having made the commitment to myself to become a yoga teacher, I also committed to attending as many training courses and events as possible to layer my knowledge and continue giving back.

I went to another module in Canberra in September and found a little more comfort in the support role.

In November there were two new courses starting in Australia, one in Melbourne and one Adelaide (both for the first time), in addition to the courses in progress in Sydney and Canberra.

I knew people in both Melbourne and Adelaide from my training course so went on the net and checked airfares. Melbourne was cheaper so I booked in to help on the Melbourne and arranged my accommodation.

Of course, as the confluence of events often happens, I was also asked to give a talk at the *Taking Control* group in Canberra on the same weekend. Not wanting to say no to either opportunity and feeling like there was something to be gained by going to both, I booked my flights to go to Melbourne on the Wednesday night and to return to Canberra on the Friday night so I could attend two days at the first Melbourne module and speak to the *Taking Control* meeting.

I was picked up at the airport by my meditation buddy's daughter, who drove me directly to her father's house in the black of night referring only to the venue as 'not far away'. I hadn't been to Melbourne for about twenty years and never driven in the city, but on the first day of the module I woke up not knowing where I was or where I was going, only knowing the name of the venue, location of the car and the car keys my friend was lending me, and that he said there was a street directory in the car.

Not very long ago I would have felt defeated, but after the last few months, I looked upon this as just another adventure. I began in my usual way of sitting in meditation and rose from my cushion with serenity and focus: 'of course I can do this'.

I found the keys and went out to the car. Now, for the last few years, we had old cars and I wasn't used to remote locking so of course the first thing that happened was I put the key in the lock and opened the door and the alarm went off... very loudly. I pushed every button on the key until the alarm stopped.

Not a great start, but I laughed at the absurdity of my situation and carried on; I wasn't going to be stopped that easily. I found the street directory and went back inside.

Next problem, I realised I didn't know the street name or the house number. There was bound to be something lying around with the address on it. A brief search of tabletops turned up an envelope with my friend's name and address – bingo.

OK, now I had everything I needed and spent the next fifteen minutes getting a bird's eye view of the general route then a more detailed street name kind of route but had no idea how long it would take to drive. I decided to dress and leave, with the street directory open on the passenger seat.

The drive through the edge of Melbourne was beautiful; houses dotted through a rural landscape with increasing density into urban. I used my usual driving breathing techniques to maintain the calm that had begun with my earlier practice and arrived in my destination suburb with plenty of time to spare, feeling triumphant.

Beware of hubris!

Traffic jam; it took as long to travel the short distance along the road to the venue as it did to get to this point. Breathing again. I called the organisers and told them I would be late and relaxed, wondering if teaching drivers to meditate when we teach them to drive would reduce the incidence of road rage.

Finally I arrived for two days of yoga and meeting yet another group of trainee yogis, some of whom have since become close friends.

Over the two days I realised two things: one, I felt really comfortable in this environment, like I belonged somehow; and two, that I had something to offer that was valuable yet different because of how I had practiced yoga.

There were many conversations during those two days on how to visualise, and how to start a practice amidst illness and busyness, and several people mentioned how moved they had been by my story and that it had been a factor of their decision to do the course. And, "you should write a book about this" (wish I had a dollar for every person who has said that over the last few years).

Next, it was back to Canberra to begin preparing for my talk at the MS Society.

Taking Control of MS is the name of a book written by George Jelinek, a man who was diagnosed with MS in the middle of a busy medical career and equally busy family life. He carried out a worldwide search for alternative approaches to living with MS out of which *Taking Control* was born. As the book circulated through Australia (and then overseas), small groups of people with MS formed to support each other in implementing the approach described in the book.

I had made contact with the Canberra group at the MS Society's Wellness Day back in May – an expo of alternative approaches to wellbeing in the local area in the morning and talks about nutrition and research in the afternoon. I was one of three yogis in a group teaching Dru yoga, and told aspects of my story and tips that had helped me through my journey with MS.

Many of the participants were shocked to see a person with MS looking so well, let alone someone who had been in a wheelchair.

Later during the talks I sat with comfort in the lotus position with a straight back, just because I had found it was the most comfortable way for me to sit, particularly for a long period. Several people noticed me sitting in this way and at the end of the talks I spoke with the organiser of the *Taking Control* group, who asked if I would come and speak to the group. I wasn't sure what I could possibly offer but agreed anyway.

In the week before the meeting I met with the organiser, David, to discuss the order of the meetings and what resources are available. I had toyed with doing a presentation, but after talking with David realised that what he actually wanted was to know why I was walking not wheeling. He just wanted to hear my story.

After discarding the idea of a presentation, I thought, 'I can't spend two hours talking about myself', and decided to teach some yoga after my talk. As the date of the talk drew nearer I spent a great deal of time thinking about what I would say and how I would say it, but I couldn't bring myself to actually write a speech.

A certain arrogance arose that 'it was my story, I've lived it, so I should be able to talk about it', which combined with a certain lack of time and a mental block whenever I even thought about writing a speech. I would just have to fly by the seat of my pants, again, and trust that what I said would be the right thing to say.

The yoga was the same as the speech; I knew the ball park of what I wanted to teach, it was embedded in my being, and I would trust what came into my head on the day. I prepared a modified EBR1 and a relaxation, in my mind.

I suspect the real reason I had not been able to write a speech for that day was a deep fear that finally I would be revealed and thus they would think me a fraud. Underneath I still didn't think I had anything extraordinary to offer and they would be left wondering why David had summoned this flaky woman to present at their meeting; 'They', being the members of the group.

I woke on Saturday morning and as usual there were still things to be done with my children, driving, shopping and feeding, so there was little time to dwell or get too nervous, but as I parked my car at the MS Society, this was the feeling in the pit of my stomach.

Again, I thanked Dru and Andrew and Trish as I used the techniques of relaxation and meditation to calm this fear and sense of inadequacy. At some point Trish had advised me to place my teachers around the room and ask for guidance, and while I wasn't sure how this would work, I figured I needed all the help I could get so did it anyway.

The members of the group arrived and sat in the semi-circle of chairs David and I had arranged, and after a brief introduction, I was on. I suddenly felt quite naked and small in front of this group of a dozen people with MS; leggings, a long sleeved t-shirt, no make-up and my hair back in a scrunchy.

"Maybe I should have written a speech, maybe I should have dressed up a little more", I mulled over as I realised I had never actually done anything like this before.

I looked to the corners of the room where I had *placed* Trish and Andrew and began. It took about an hour to tell my story, up to standing there on the day. Wow, I didn't think I had that much to say. During my talk everyone was very quiet and respectful, but aside from the audience being polite, I found it impossible to gauge the response.

'Did they think I was a wanker?'

After I finished talking, I asked if they wanted to do some yoga and they unanimously agreed. Phew, comfort zone! I knew I could teach yoga. We did a quick warm-up and then the first half of EBR1. I looked around and it was time for a break so we paused while everyone got a drink.

Smiling, chatting, that looks good.

Everyone seemed keen to continue, so I finished EBR1, then I guided them through a therapy massaging each other's shoulders so they could see how easy it was to offer comfort, followed by a brief relaxation. Two hours goes quite quickly, really.

At the end I offered to do a regular class or short course if anyone was interested, thanked them,and

David closed the meeting. I think those moments when I began to pack up my mat were as difficult as any during the previous 2½ hours, like the moments after a performance between finishing and (hopefully) applause – did they like it or not?

The response was unanimously positive. Thank god! One by one people approached me to thank me for sharing my story and teaching yoga; apparently my story was inspiring and the yoga left their bodies feeling good and relaxed. In addition, most were interested in taking classes in some form.

Perhaps they didn't think I was a wanker or a fraud.

Then two very special things happened. First, a woman who had been sitting in the back on a scooter approached me. When I was talking about my surrender she had an epiphany that that was what she needed to do; she had been angry and fighting and she needed to surrender. I gave her my number and later we arranged ongoing one-on-one sessions. She has become a close friend and is now learning how to surrender.

Later, I was talking to a lady in a wheelchair about the last few months of her life, which hadn't been easy, and she said, "But I was nowhere as sick as you were". At the time I dismissed it as untrue, 'I wasn't that sick'.

Then at some point about an hour later as I was driving down to Braidwood to pick up Nicola, I felt completely overwhelmed by a sudden wave of realisation that she was right. I had been that sick.

I pulled over as the wave of realisation became a wave of emotion and I sat at the wheel of my car sobbing until it was done. For the first time I deeply understood the magnitude of my journey over the last six years and I have never felt such gratitude; gratitude for my teachers, for my practice and the love I had received that enabled me to share my story.

After everyone but David had left the room, I thanked my teachers in the corners of the room and released the thought. It had been comforting to have them there. Thanked David who was beaming and has also become a close friend, and left.

The confluence of these events was not coinciden-tal, they taught me different aspects of the same lesson: the story of my journey was inspiring to people who have MS and people who don't; people do want to hear it; my experiences have given something special to offer as a yoga teacher even to able-bodied people; and that maybe I'm not a fraud.

The Essence Was Trust

NOVEMBER/DECEMBER 2009

In the months immediately after the initial emotional turmoil of separation, Matthew and I established calm between us. We were both determined to put the children's interests first and maintain at least a civil relationship and I think we both wanted to preserve our friendship – we had shared the most significant moments of our lives together for the last 17½ years and wanted to respect our history.

However, tension was coming into our calm, threatening to bring storm and turmoil back into our smooth sea– the property settlement. My inclination was to chill but I was receiving support to be more aggressive; it played on my financially insecure position and the underlying lack of safety I felt.

I thought we were keeping it between us but children are antennae for tension and I had started to notice my youngest playing out our conflict; she just wasn't like that. Then on the way home from work one day I struck every red light on the drive. (I usually use red lights as an opportunity to do some pranayama and connect with my higher self a little or ask difficult questions.)

For example, why was Nicola behaving in this way?

Almost immediately I realised her behaviour was a reflection of the tension that had developed between her parents. That was the first couple of red lights.

Then over the next couple I realised the most important lesson: I did not need to be paid to have been married to Matthew, I had done so out of love and I felt love. I wasn't owed anything by anyone.

The only debt was from us to our children to provide them with material wellbeing and emotional security, none of which was going to happen if we continued to create tension over money. I resolved to call Matthew that evening and attempt to resolve the discord.

It didn't happen immediately but it did happen and we had a financial agreement signed and sorted by Christmas, and on Christmas Eve I bought myself my first car.

The essence was trust and I trusted him completely to look after the children as well as he could, and once he understood my willingness to let go, he could also relax.

Anaphylaxis

DECEMBER 2009

The first six weeks of my drug regime went swimmingly. I felt less fatigued and the side effects were more pronounced than when I started the injections but they were manageable. I had no problem with the injections and was even able to manually inject.

Then the swellings at the sites of injection became larger and took longer to recede; and the pain at the time of injection was also getting worse and also took longer to recede. I thought it was perhaps my imagination but the swellings were starting to still be present when the cycle returned and for that time they had been tender.

I continued.

If it worsened I would go back to the doctor.

Then one sunny morning in December, I sat as usual for meditation and injection. Everything was the same as it had been every other morning for the last two months. As soon as the fluid was injected I knew there was something wrong; the pain was excruciating at the site of injection, and an ice-cold, slightly metallic feeling immediately shot to my brain.

I started to feel the urge to throw up and pass diarrhoea simultaneously so I scuttled to the toilet. I started to sweat and feel dizzy, and my lips started to swell. I could hardly walk the short distance to my room and lay down at my altar. My throat started to swell and I was having difficulty breathing.

I was still chanting, as was my practice, and trying to relax; I thought I was going to die. My eldest daughter came in to see if I was alright and I asked her to get the Ventolin we had for Nicola's brief period of asthma earlier in the year. I took the Ventolin and waited; if I couldn't breathe soon I would have to call an ambulance. Everything was starting to tingle and I felt very sleepy.

Finally my breathing started to ease and the acute phase of the reaction began to diminish. Again I started to become aware of the chant that had been going in the back of my mind and felt incredible relief as I started to cry.

The girls needed to get to school and I needed to get to work; I was in an altered state of consciousness. I showered and dressed and called the girls' schools. I was still crying. Crying all the way as I drove first Grace and then Nicola to school.

On the way to my school I became aware of being surrounded by a familiar but unearthly light; at one of the sets of lights I realised it was the same light I had seen with the Buddhist monk in Byron Bay.

Another wave of tears came as I realised what had happened and all the trivial things that had passed through my mind in the previous few days came again through my mind. I realised the only important thing in this life was to love; first it was my children and then all others. In that moment all I wanted was to live in that light.

I arrived at work with a swollen face and nausea at the edge, with the threat of a headache hanging over my awareness. All day I meditated and breathed to keep the panic (and the symptoms) at bay. I tried to contact both my neurologist and my GP without success. I still wasn't sure whether to take my injection the next day or even what had actually happened.

And in the background of every breath was my desire to live as an expression of the light.

I looked up anaphylactic reaction on the internet and my symptoms seemed to fit but I wasn't sure because I had never had one. Soon after I arrived home I received a call from the neurology nurse and was told under no circumstances take another dose, and yes, I had had an anaphylactic reaction that probably should been attended by a health professional. Oops.

I still had running around to do, to get Grace to the school play, pick up Nicola and take her to Grace's school play, and then to the Dru office for a meeting. Finally I arrived at home, exhausted at about 9.30pm.

The day had passed in a surreal state of shock,

meditation and light. I had moved from one responsibility to another with only the energy provided by being in absolute surrender and presence; with the understanding that in reality the only meaning came from the love I felt and the love I gave.

It took quite a while to recover from this reaction as it brought on a mild relapse in the days that followed, but after a week or so I was back to where I was before the reaction.

When first discussing the different drug regimes and side effects with my neurologist, I stressed I didn't want to try any drug with depression as a side effect. I have experienced clinical depression and I have grown up with depression and I would rather be in a wheelchair. In a wheelchair I can laugh and love my children but with depression I can't do any of that.

The neurologist stressed it wasn't about just the mobility, but loss of my hands and my cognitive abilities. I had experienced all of these and still would prefer this to depression. I could love without all of these functions and that was what was important.

Soon after this I resolved to manage MS, drug-free. I don't regret the decision to begin drug treatment and don't want this to be used to push drug-free management regimes. I know many people who have years of incident-free drug treatment behind them, but for me I will risk trusting yoga and meditation.

Surrender

A friend of mine recently asked, "How do I surrender? I know I need to but how do you do it?"

It was a difficult question to answer because it was something that just seemed to happen for me. I had never taken any notice of how it happened, only that it did. I knew the difference in state of mind and the impact it has had on my every-day life but not the 'how to' route or indeed what surrender actually is.

Then one night, deep in meditation, I discovered what surrender was (at least for me) and then possibly how to get there, consciously.

I think surrender is a deep physical and energetic relaxation to what is; and therefore, the path to surrender is paved with relaxation and begins with regular physical relaxation.

I found that resistance expresses itself in me in the form of tightness; physical, mental and/or emotional.

Physically, it might be the way I am holding my body, shallow or constricted breathing or tightness in a particular part of the body.

I can be holding myself tightly while standing or sitting, have clenched jaw without being aware, tightness in my chest, holding on with my toes or my hands, holding my tummy in or holding tension in my shoulders.

Emotionally I can be feeling angry, depressed, envious, deprived, lonely or wanting.

Mentally I can be stuck in a cycle of thoughts, thinking about what might have been, what could be or projection.

Or any combination of the above.

In my experience both mental and emotional tightness will be expressed somewhere in my body and physical tightness is usually an expression of emotional or mental tightness i.e. resistance. So, working on one will undoubtedly work through the other levels of my being.

From the beginning of my yoga teaching training I have trained myself to scan my body regularly to find where I am holding tension, having seen the advantage of relaxation while in hospital after Module 1.

I could be in the middle of a public place or at home in the kitchen and notice tension in my hands or feet, and consciously use my outgoing breath to relax that part of my body. When I began driving again, I constantly relaxed through my body and mind to reduce the fatigue of driving any distance. (see **Tips for releasing tension** p.364)

So, while I was training myself to relax through doctors' appointments, examinations, tests and scans, I was inadvertently training my mind to surrender to what is. Surrendering wasn't a wham-bam-thank-you-maam, all in one hit thing; it was a gradual process of relaxing my energy system.

I consciously used my breath to breathe tension out of my body when I was in difficult situations and the more I did it the easier and more spontaneous it became. It is now automatic to change the pattern of my breath in a crisis situation; I do it without thinking about it, in fact before thinking.

Really, pranayama is just moving energy around the body with the breath, and you can do that even with limited lung capacity – it's the awareness that makes the difference.

I have found that once you learn how to relax in the privacy of your own home when you have space and time, and you do it regularly, it is a small step to taking it into the context of your everyday life so you can relax when you really need it. Eventually your body and mind just know what to do, almost automatically. (see *a quick relaxation you can do anywhere, anytime in any posture* p.364)

Sometimes I still have to be reminded by my teachers to walk at the pace of my heart or just allow myself to be, but increasingly the state of surrender is my natural state, and if I find myself resisting, surrender is just a thought and a breath away.

The times of greatest surrender in my life have

been underpinned by a deep sense of relaxation, a deep letting go of how things should be and acceptance of how things are.

Tips for releasing tension

I once had a yoga teacher who would take us into a posture and then ask us to relax our toes because many of us were holding on with our toes. I still find this invaluable advice. Since then, Dru teachers have drawn my attention to thumbs and necks – equally invaluable. These little triggers can really help to keep your body and mind to stay soft in so many situations

If my neck, toes and thumbs are relaxed, then my body-posture is usually relaxed and this instantly brings softness to my mind.

Softening my gaze is also an instant trigger to my emotional and mental layers – relax!

A quick relaxation you can do anywhere, anytime in any posture (sitting or lying).

- *Gently close your eyes, keeping them soft.*
- *Beginning with your toes, create a wave of tension with the in-breath.*
- *Relax the body, from the toes up, with the out-breath.*
- *Repeat this wave of tensing and relaxing a few times until the body is relaxed.*
- *Breathe warmth in through your toes, into*

your feet, flowing up into your ankles. Allow
the warmth to soothe any tension it finds.

- With each breath take this warmth further
and further into your body; your legs, into
your abdomen, chest, hands, arms, shoulders,
neck and head.

- Allow the warmth to rest in your heart and
sit with this still warmth for a few moments.

- When you are ready to come back to your
daily life, imagine a brilliant light above your
head radiating vibrancy and wellbeing.

- Again using the breath, draw that brilliance
into your body, through your crown, into
your arms, chest, abdomen, hips, legs and out
through your feet.

- Imagine your body waking up and becoming
more vibrant as the light moves through.

- Stretch your arms and legs, rub your hands
together and place your palms over your
closed eyes.

- Open your eyes into the warm, velvety darkness of your palms and begin gently massaging your scalp and face.

- Take a few breaths to really wake up before returning to your day and remember this
feeling of relaxation.

Naught Kinder Than Folk

One of the great gifts for me in writing this book has been the opportunity to revisit the many moments of kindness and friendship I have been privileged to experience through the events I have described and thereby reframe a belief I have held as long as I can remember.

The belief I have held so deeply through much of my life is that people wouldn't like me, and that particularly in groups I would be on the outside: hurt, ostracised and bullied. That people would find me boring, and even if they liked me initially, would see through me and eventually turn away.

Even when I wheeled into my first yoga module I expected not to be liked. Yet as I have written and read through these pages, I have realised I can no longer hold this belief with any authenticity.

There have been so many acts of random kindness,

carers who have become friends, a counsellor who believed in me and supported me, mentoring relationships with people such as Trish and Andrew that have yielded such depth and connection and a trust I didn't think was possible; and not to forget the camaraderie between and with my yoga/meditation that is the essence of life.

A young professional woman in my yoga course who seems (and is) incredibly competent sought out my company and counsel, and has now become a close friend. A man in my meditation course with many more years of experience in yoga and meditation than I may ever have has befriended me as an equal.

My experience of my relationships with my family – my children, Matthew and my siblings – has been transformed. No longer the resentful runt of the family, I feel like I belong. My children are gorgeous and Matthew and I are close friends.

I have hosted yoga and meditation 'sleepovers', formed invaluable and deep connections with my teachers and enjoyed friendship at a level I had never imagined possible for me. For someone who wasn't very good at relationships, I now seem to find friendship and kindness wherever I go with whoever I meet.

I am often astounded by people's generosity of spirit and willingness to put themselves on the line for others.

And I smile, all the time.

So what has changed?

I now look for reasons to like people. I now look

for the goodness in people and for what's common between us. I want to hear people's stories and I am not afraid to look into people's eyes. I am not afraid of people's dark bits any more.

Why? Because I'm not afraid of my own dark bits. In my search for peace I have discovered that even my worst fears and deepest held beliefs can be transformed; and when they are faced they are not so dark and scary anyway. In making friends with myself I can now make friends with other people. I can look into their eyes because I can at last allow myself to be seen. I can befriend people because I have made friends with myself.

I have often heard and said the phrase, "naught queerer than folk", but now I think, "naught kinder than folk".

Spirituality of Healing

The spirituality of my journey with MS has been woven in through my story and so when the idea of a separate chapter on spirituality came to me, I wondered why. Then I started to think about the healing journeys that have inspired me through these last few years (Petrea King, Ian Gawler, George Jelinek, The Journey and Lance Armstrong), and I realised they all have a spiritual component, so it must be worth exploring. So I'll just write and see what happens.

When I read back through the pages of my story, the significant moments for me have occurred within the context of experiencing an extraordinary sense of peace; a peace so vast and so deep as to absorb any mitigating circumstances like drops in the ocean. These have also been the moments of the deepest healing of the emotional and psychological pain that has plagued me all my life.

The experience of peace is what I now call spirituality and the techniques I use to bring about that sense of peace are what I call my spiritual practices. It's really no more oobey-goobey than that.

What I have discovered is that the field of peace is always here, lying underneath the clutter of everyday life, and the more I practice the more easily I can access the field and thus the more I experience it. And the more I experience peace, the better my life is and the lives of those around me because it is within the context of that deep nurturing, soothing sense of peace our minds can rest and in which healing occurs.

And that's why it's so important for healing journeys to have a spiritual component, not only because being in this state of mind is more pleasant but also because it expands our vision beyond the immediate physical reality into something bigger. The life of someone with a chronic illness can become so myopic, and so connecting with this deep field of peace in us all enables us to see ourselves in perspective, connected with others around us.

For me it has been the primary motivator. It is also what led me to Dru; not because I hoped to find peace in Dru but because I experienced it most when I practiced Dru. The smallest practices would give me a taste of peace; change the feeling in my mind just a little bit to expand my vision beyond what I was feeling, particularly beyond what I was lacking.

So rather than focussing on what I had lost or the physical discomfort I experienced by having a chronic illness, I started to think about how I could give; not because I'm a hero but because it's a natural consequence of feeling peace.

Learning how to access this underlying stillness is also helping me to peel away the layers of self-hate that have prevented me from true happiness in my life, and enabling me to begin learning how to fulfil my own personal goal of loving unconditionally, which to me is far more important than whether I walk or not.

So my spiritual life began with a yearning to live in the peace I came upon by accident while feeling like a big bag of excrement. In practicality, it began with small random practices that resonated with me (a fancy new-age term meaning 'felt good'); first, the mantra of compassion from the autobiography of the Dalai Lama's sister, and reading the *Little book of Happiness* by the man himself, while practicing my hotch-potch combination of yoga and physiotherapy exercises in Britain.

Then, when I began Dru classes, it was the little things that had the most impact on my daily life: becoming aware of my posture, do-in etc. Doing these little things through my day somehow carried the energy of the class and were like drops of water wearing away at my cliff. Those drops began a revolution in the way I look at life and the way I live my life, and I am deeply grateful.

Dru is a discipline of yoga and so is based in the Vedic traditions. The Bhagavad Gita has been an inspiration on my journey as have the writings of the Dalai Lama but I am not a Hindu or a Buddhist. The sense of peace I am writing about is non-denominational and I have experienced it while reading about St Francis' life, Islam and other spiritual disciplines.

Through Dru, I have met a Catholic nun, Buddhists, Sanyassin yogis, shamans and new-agers, and they all describe the same sense of peace when they practice. Practitioners of tai chi and other martial arts also describe the same sense of stillness, as do meditators.

So it doesn't really matter what you call it, rather that you find a practice that does it for you and do it.

I didn't have a spontaneous awakening or sit under a tree or go on a self discovery odyssey or even a spiritual pilgrimage and the closest I came to retreat were the four-day modules, where I learned how to teach yoga and meditation. I sat in my lounge room or on a bus, at work or in the kitchen or a hospital room, with my kids and without, and I practiced peace.

The diagnosis of a chronic illness, whether terminal or not is life changing, and dealing with it calls for nothing less than changing your life. In my own experience of both struggle and acceptance, acceptance is by far the easier path, and developing a spiritual practice facilitates embracing acceptance and that has made my life better than it was before, with or without MS.

That's why I had to write the chapter.

So What Does My Story Mean?

As I come to the close of this chapter of my journey I am wondering how my story will be interpreted by those who read it.

I am aware there are sceptics who will not give any significance to my yoga and meditation practice and dismiss my recovery as just another chapter in the story of MS – the mystery disease, nothing more remarkable than a spontaneous remission.

There are those who will say it's a miracle or that I must be extraordinary.

So now I ask to ask myself.

"How do I interpret my journey? What does it mean for me?"

The honest answer is that I believe I am reconfiguring my energy system. For two and a half years I have devoted most of my daily thoughts to striving for the highest I was capable of at the time. I have used the power of my mind to visualise yoga, meditate, chant ancient mantras of light, relax and transform my daily experience of life.

I haven't been perfect. I have made mistakes in the way I relate to people and community; I have been very human, and these moments of perceived failure have caused me excruciating emotional pain. What I have done is maintain the original intention to move toward freedom and that intention planted the seed for a tree of transformation that is still growing.

I have practiced every day, sometimes all day and all night; eating, cooking, watching TV, interacting with my children, waiting in queues, on public transport, in my car, in hospital beds, at rock concerts, at work and at home.

It's not a miracle in the sense that I went to sleep one day and woke up cured the next; and I'm not extraordinary in the sense of being particularly gifted in any way. I have just worked very hard.

The techniques I have used are based in ancient practice and anyone can learn to use them.

What I've learnt from my practice is that everything the body does is sending messages to your mind and everything your mind does is sending messages to your body and spirit. The mind, body and spirit are in constant interaction.

In a balanced and integrated system, this interaction is harmonic, producing a beautiful composition called wellbeing, which I've also discovered doesn't necessarily mean injury or disability free. We have all heard of people with permanent disability, chronic illness or sometimes even terminal illness who radiate wellness; and I have even experienced it myself. It simply means, within the constraints of their physical condition, that person has found harmony and balance.

My goal was peace of mind, and so bit by bit I have dismantled limiting beliefs and thought patterns, each time finding renewed physical wellbeing.

I haven't cured MS. Every day I experience symptoms to remind me of the damage to my CNS, but I have cleared away years of accumulated emotional debris, enabling me to access the world of energy beyond material structure.

When I began, I didn't expect to get out of my wheelchair let alone do cartwheels, and as my relapse in 2009 has shown me, I am still a breath away from returning. The peace I found while in a wheelchair, in a hospital bed and now on legs, is accessible to anyone who is willing to spend some time each day in stillness and surrender to the circumstances of their lives, as they are.

The most valuable consequence of my journey into stillness is the effect it has on the people around me, most noticeably my children. I have been taught when any individual takes a step toward their own personal harmony that it will ripple out into the world around them. My experience over the last five years is an expression of this philosophy.

As I have grown, my parenting has improved. I

react less, listen more and love more. I need to be right less and give guidance only when asked, instructing less when I think they 'should'.

In the broader world, the more I accept myself and become conscious of my own dark corners and idiosyncratic behaviours, the more accepting I am of those I meet. I react less, criticise less and look at conflict as an opportunity to learn something more about myself. The result is greater harmony in my relationships with the world around me, something I feel on a daily basis.

And the most valuable gift is surrender.

Through 2009, I experienced both pain and pleasure; triumph and perceived failure. I felt a crippling envy of those who were able to go on retreat or travel to pursue their spirituality or even have a holiday; debilitating angst, anger and betrayal as well as joy and love.

But as the trees in Canberra began to grow green and the flowers to blossom, I reflected on the previous few months, almost like a witness to my own life and its outcomes, and learned what might be the most valuable lesson of my journey – deep surrender.

I have grown and learned and let go of attachments as a result of each life experience, good and bad. My peace of mind has expanded and my wellbeing deepened, and as it has all occurred in the context of my everyday life, there is no fear of it disappearing when I return to my life.

I have watched people return from retreat and seen the same light in their eyes as I have felt in my own. Their step is no lighter than my own, their love of life no greater.

Ultimately, I have realised good and bad are the same; either way we grow and learn or stagnate, depending on our attitude. I have learned, from my own experience, to look for the lesson in even the smallest of moments and feel gratitude for all experiences, and this has given me freedom from dependence on my life being perfect.

Sometimes life seems far from perfect, sometimes life just is and that's enough. My lesson is to surrender to what is; embrace what is and what happens next is joy. A little bubbling well of joy that is increasingly close to the surface, arising in the most unlikely of places.

Perhaps for me, this is the essence of my journey, a simple nine letter word beginning with s – surrender. There are no boundaries, nothing to defend, so surrender; surrender to the present and everything else vanishes.

"Letting go of everything, with your whole heart take refuge in Me, for I will free you of everything that causes you pain. There is no need for fear or worry."

My favourite verse from the Gita has become a mantra for me. I chant the Sanskrit every day. 'Me' can be God (in whatever form you worship), the void, your higher self or simply the present moment. Allow your mind to be so open and accepting of the person or the events right in front of you, that past and future yearnings become irrelevant.

Oh, and yes, I can cartwheel on a good day.

Heart meditation

This is a meditation for when you need love in your life. It is a good idea if you can do some gentle movement to reduce restlessness in your body and mind before you settle for meditation.

- *Sit or lie in a comfortable position, with your spine as straight as possible.*
- *Breathe in and contract your muscles from your toes to your crown and relax on your breath out. Repeat a few times until you are feeling relaxed.*
- *Gently close your eyes and take a few moments to notice your breathing.*
- *Become aware of your breastbone moving in and out as you breathe.*
- *Feel your heart and imagine breathing in and out of your heart.*
- *Invite your mind to remember a time in your life when you felt really loved, and if you can't remember, imagine what being loved might feel like.*
- *Allow your mind to focus on the feeling (it may evoke a sensation, colour and or sound) and let the feeling fill your awareness.*
- *Sit in that feeling for a few moments.*
- *Then, when you are ready to come out of the meditation offer the feeling to someone who may be in need of feeling loved; let it go on your breath out.*

- *Deepen you breath and notice the clothes on your skin and your weight on the chair.*
- *Rub your palms together, gently open your eyes into your warmed palms and massage your face.*
- *Take a few moments before returning to your day and appreciate the stillness and love you have found in your own heart.*

What now?

Since the beginning of 2010 I have experienced MS exacerbations with heat, sleep deprivation, writing this book and busyness. Every day I feel the symptoms of the illness that has taken me to a wheelchair three times.

I haven't cured MS.

Yet no symptom is overwhelming, no exacerbation lasts for more than a couple of days, if that. My system seems to have learned how to come back on line and when my movements lose the feeling of smoothness most of us associate with moving, I use my mind to find it again; I use my mind to find my function and/ or find another route.

I now use yoga and meditation to manage MS, and every other aspect of my life; and teach yoga, relaxation and meditation to people from four years old to 64, with MS, cancer and autism, as well as people without disability.

When my tai chi teacher told me I could visualise movement in 2004, I couldn't get my head around it but I let the evidence of my body, and other peoples', speak for itself. When my yoga teachers told me I could visualise yoga, I still didn't quite believe them but I wanted peace.

Now having spent the last four years learning yoga practices to move energy around my body, I just move the energy around my body with my mind.

I have discovered the value and importance of deep relaxation at every level of my being, which underlies surrender – not in the least a passive process.

I started my search as a search for peace; to learn how to live in peace and to learn how to share peace. What I have found is that peace is a natural state of mind resting underneath, waiting for us to relax long enough to be present, even through difficult life circumstances; and sharing peace is simply a matter of living peace.

And what I have experienced is but a spark of the splendour...

"Wherever you see anything that is beautiful, glorious and mighty, know that it springs from a mere spark of My essence and splendour."

- The Dru Bhagavad Gita, chapter 10, verse 41

What is Dru?

Dru is a lineage of yoga and meditation named after the Sanskrit term for the North Star, representing eternal stillness. This is what we seek in every Dru practice – the stillness at the heart of all action and the action within all stillness.

DRU CONTACTS:

Dru Australia
Australian Dru Yoga Office
4 Pandanus Street, Fisher, ACT 2611
Tel: (02) 6161 1462
Fax: 02 6287 7480
E: info@dru.com.au
website: www.dru.com.au

Dru Worldwide
Snowdonia Mountain Lodge
Nant Ffrancon
Bethesda, Bangor
LL57 3LX
E: hello@druworldwide.com
T: 01248 602900
F: 01248 602004
website: www.druworldwide.con

Dru Australia courses
Dru Yoga Teacher Training Course
Dru Meditation Teacher Training Course
Dru Post-Graduate Mastery Course
There are many Dru seminars and retreats offered in Australia and overseas so if you are interested, please go to the Dru websites and find the next event near you.
Dru Tips for Life, a regular email newsletter offering yoga and meditation tips to use in every-day life, can be accessed via the Dru Australia website.

		QTY
Journey to Peace Through Yoga	$26.99	....
Postage within Australia (1 book)	$5.00	....
Postage within Australia (2 or more books)	$9.00	....

TOTAL* $_____

* All prices include GST

Name: ....

Address: ....

....

Phone: ....

Email Address: ....

Payment:

❏ Money Order ❏ Cheque ❏ Amex ❏ MasterCard ❏ Visa

Cardholder's Name:..

Credit Card Number: ....

Signature:...

Expiry Date: ....

Allow 21 days for delivery.

Payment to: Better Bookshop (ABN 14 067 257 390)
PO Box 12544
A'Beckett Street, Melbourne, 8006
Victoria, Australia
betterbookshop@brolgapublishing.com.au

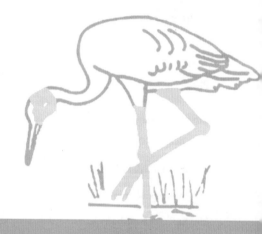

BE PUBLISHED

Publishing through a successful Australian publisher. Brolga provides:

- Editorial appraisal
- Cover design
- Typesetting
- Printing
- Author promotion
- National book trade distribution, including sales, marketing and distribution through Macmillan Australia.

For details and inquiries, contact:
Brolga Publishing Pty Ltd
PO Box 12544
A'Beckett St VIC 8006

Phone: 03 9600 4982
bepublished@brolgapublishing.com.au
markzocchi@brolgapublishing.com.au
ABN: 46 063 962 443